Carotid Artery Disease: Surgical Perspectives

Djordje Radak • Stevo Duvnjak
Editors

Carotid Artery Disease: Surgical Perspectives

Springer

Editors
Djordje Radak
Serbian Academy of Sciences and Arts
Belgrade, Serbia

Stevo Duvnjak
Department of Vascular Surgery
Rigshospitalet
Copenhagen, Denmark

ISBN 978-3-031-81841-7 ISBN 978-3-031-81842-4 (eBook)
https://doi.org/10.1007/978-3-031-81842-4

This Springer imprint is published by the registered company Springer Nature Switzerland AG
The registered company address is: Gewerbestrasse 11, 6330 Cham, Switzerland

"A man is infinitely more complicated than his thoughts"

– Paul Valery

"I do not believe in things. I believe in relationships"

– Georges Braque

Preface

Carotid surgery is a frequently performed operation that brings great satisfaction to both patients and surgeons. Supra-aortic artery disease is managed through open and endovascular surgery, benefiting our patients and preventing severe complications that could arise if left untreated. This book aims to provide residents and young vascular surgeons with a quick overview of carotid and subclavian artery diseases, covering the diagnosis and surgical decision-making processes. By focusing on this specific topic within vascular surgery, readers can gain up-to-date knowledge, from diagnosis to treatment.

The book introduces the reader to supra-aortic vessel diseases and includes brief but important historical facts about the courageous pioneers and developments in vascular surgery. Clinical examination, diagnosis, conservative management, open surgery, and endovascular treatment are discussed in separate chapters. The authors, who are experienced in both open and endovascular treatments of supra-aortic arteries, hope this book will serve as a practical overview. Other surgical colleagues and medical students may also find this book useful.

The Editors would like to thank the contributing authors and welcome any suggestions or comments.

Belgrade, Serbia
Copenhagen, Denmark
2024

Djordje Radak
Stevo Duvnjak

Contents

Contributors

Goetz Benndorf, MD, PhD Professor, Department of Radiology, Baylor College of Medicine, One Baylor Plaza, Houston, TX, USA

Stevo Duvnjak Department of Vascular Surgery, Rigshospitalet, Copenhagen, Denmark

Jes S. Lindholt Department of Cardiothoracic and Vascular Surgery, Odense University Hospital, Odense, Denmark

Djordje Radak Serbian Academy of Sciences and Arts, Belgrade, Serbia

Clinic for Surgery, Euromedik Hospital, Belgrade, Serbia

Introduction

1

Djordje Radak and Stevo Duvnjak

The carotid arteries are the blood vessels that supply the brain. Although the brain constitutes only 2–3% of an adult's body mass, it receives about 20% of the blood output from the heart and utilizes up to 25% of the oxygen and 20% of the glucose from systemic circulation [1]. Cerebrovascular diseases are conditions in which pathological processes damage one or more blood vessels in the brain, leading to temporary or permanent damage from ischemia or bleeding.

1.1 Introduction

- 80% of cerebrovascular diseases are ischemic
- while 20% result from hemorrhage [2]

Cerebrovascular disease is the third leading cause of death, the second leading cause of dementia, and the most common cause of disability worldwide [3]. In Europe, Serbia ranks second in stroke frequency, particularly among women. Insufficient blood supply to the brain is responsible for 60–70% of cases, primarily due to diseases of the carotid arteries, which are treatable. Atherosclerotic narrowing is a common cause, but other carotid artery diseases are increasingly being recognized. For patients who experience a transient ischemic attack (TIA) and exhibit initial symptoms of brain malnutrition, the risk of a subsequent stroke is

D. Radak
Serbian Academy of Sciences and Arts, Belgrade, Serbia

Clinic for Surgery, Euromedik Hospital, Belgrade, Serbia
e-mail: radak@ikvbd.com

S. Duvnjak (✉)
Department of Vascular Surgery, Rigshospitalet, Copenhagen, Denmark
e-mail: stevo.duvnjak@regionh.dk

D. Radak, S. Duvnjak (eds.), *Carotid Artery Disease: Surgical Perspectives*,
https://doi.org/10.1007/978-3-031-81842-4_1

approximately 5–11% within the first year [4]. This risk is even higher for those who have already had a stroke. The medical, familial, social, and economic consequences of cerebrovascular diseases are severe. Carotid disease accounts for about 70% of ischemic stroke cases, yet it is the only cause that can be effectively and reliably treated through revascularization.

The objectives of carotid reconstruction—whether through endarterectomy, bypass, or stenting—are to prevent ischemic stroke, alleviate neurological symptoms and complaints, and possibly prevent vascular dementia, cognitive disorders, and senility. A successful arterial reconstruction requires both:

- **Wisdom in determining indications**
- **Precision in the technical execution of the procedure**

The brain is the organ through which we learn, influence the world, and change ourselves. Carotid disease impairs brain nutrition, leading to neurological and neuropsychological damage. The functioning of the central nervous system is dependent on adequate blood flow through the brain.

The bloodstream supplies the brain with oxygen and glucose, essential for energy production, as well as amino acids, which are precursors for neurotransmitters and other substances necessary for synthesizing functional molecules to maintain brain homeostasis. Circulation also removes metabolic waste from the brain. Neurons, the basic units of brain function, form a complex network of synaptic communications responsible for sensory, motor, autonomic, cognitive, and emotional functions. Damage to nerve cells caused by insufficient nutrition is mostly irreversible.

Vascular dementia, or cognitive and vascular deterioration, is poised to become a significant global challenge in the coming century.

The substantial increase in life expectancy means that more people are living beyond 80 years, during which time atherosclerotic lesions progressively develop. Chronic brain ischemia does not always result in an acute stroke, but each episode that worsens the degree of chronic ischemia—conditions to which these individuals have often adapted—leads to further irreversible loss of neuronal function and their synaptic networks. The saying "The brain does not complain, nor does it forgive" aptly reflects this phenomenon.

Prolonged chronic malnutrition of the brain may not necessarily lead to an acute stroke, but it can cause macro- and micro-lacunar lesions, leading to brain atrophy and deterioration of fine brain functions, including neurological, neuropsychological, emotional, endocrine, and regulatory functions [5]. Once irreversible brain damage occurs, revascularization is of no benefit.

Stroke has significant social, emotional, and economic consequences for individuals, families, and society. Early diagnosis and treatment of brain ischemia, particularly related to carotid disease, are hindered by public awareness. Many people are unaware that carotid disease is the only cause of stroke that can be reliably treated with a relatively safe and straightforward intervention. Moreover, because brain ischemia often does not cause pain, patients may ignore or downplay their symptoms. For many years, these interventions were considered risky. However, extensive clinical studies conducted at the end of the last century conclusively demonstrated the benefits of brain revascularization [6, 7].

References

1. Erbsloh F, Bernsmeier A, Hillesheim H. Der Glucoseverbrauch des Gehirns und seine Abhängigkeit von der Leber [The brain glucose consumption & its dependence on the liver]. Arch Psychiatr Nervenkr Z Gesamte Neurol Psychiatr. 1958;196:611–26.
2. Davis SM, Donnan GA. Clinical practice. Secondary prevention after ischemic stroke or transient ischemic attack. N Engl J Med. 2012;366:1914–22.
3. Go AS, Mozaffarian D, Roger VL, Benjamin EJ, Berry JD, Blaha MJ, et al. Heart disease and stroke statistics—2014 update: a report from the American Heart Association. Circulation. 2014;129:e28–292.
4. Giles MF, Rothwell PM. Risk of stroke early after transient ischaemic attack: a systematic review and meta-analysis. Lancet Neurol. 2007;6:1063–72.
5. Leung KKG, Bartlett JW, Barnes J, Manning EN, Ourselin S, Fox NC, Alzheimer's Disease Neuroimaging Initiative. Cerebral atrophy in mild cognitive impairment and Alzheimer disease: rates and acceleration. Neurology. 2013;80:648–54.
6. European Carotid Surgery Trialists' Collaborative Group. Randomised trial of endarterectomy for recently symptomatic carotid stenosis: final results of the MRC European carotid surgery trial (ECST). Lancet. 1998;351:1379–87.
7. North American Symptomatic Carotid Endarterectomy Trial Collaborators. The beneficial effect of carotid endarterectomy in symptomatic patients with high-grade carotid stenosis. N Engl J Med. 1991;325:445–53.

Relevant Historical Facts

2

Djordje Radak and Stevo Duvnjak

The word "carotid" is derived from the Greek word "karos," meaning "to sink into a deep sleep" [1]. In Latin, they were called *arteriae soporales* or "arteries of sleep." Compression of the carotid artery can cause temporary loss of consciousness. For centuries, the cause of stroke was unknown and often considered "God's punishment." It was not understood that the brain is nourished through the carotid arteries, so the idea that these arteries could be the cause of a stroke was not considered.

Galen (131–201 AD) discovered through animal dissections that arteries contain blood and deduced that blood nourishes the brain [1].

Virchow (1856) observed a connection between carotid thrombosis and brain ischemia, which could result in blindness [2].

Chiari (1905) reported that thrombotic deposits at the base of carotid plaques cause embolization of cerebral arteries, leading to stroke [3].

Carrel (1905) published seminal work on the technique of arterial anastomoses in animal experiments, laying the foundation for vascular and transplantation surgery, for which he later received the Nobel Prize [4].

Takayasu (1908) identified arteritis of the brachiocephalic arteries (manifesting as absent pulsations in the neck arteries) as the cause of ischemic retinal lesions [5].

Hunt (1914) was the first to publish evidence that carotid artery thrombosis leads to ischemic cerebral infarction and contralateral hemiplegia [6].

D. Radak
Serbian Academy of Sciences and Arts, Belgrade, Serbia

Clinic for Surgery, Euromedik Hospital, Belgrade, Serbia
e-mail: radak@ikvbd.com

S. Duvnjak (✉)
Department of Vascular Surgery, Rigshospitalet, Copenhagen, Denmark
e-mail: stevo.duvnjak@regionh.dk

D. Radak, S. Duvnjak (eds.), *Carotid Artery Disease: Surgical Perspectives*,
https://doi.org/10.1007/978-3-031-81842-4_2

Egas Moniz (1937) developed the technique of cerebral arteriography in Portugal, for which he was later awarded the Nobel Prize for his work on prefrontal leucotomy [7].

Miller Fisher (1941) demonstrated the correlation between pathological findings in the carotid arteries and cerebral ischemia, distinguishing between the hemodynamic and emboligenic consequences of carotid atherosclerotic plaques [8].

DeBakey (1953), the world-renowned surgeon of Lebanese origin, performed the first carotid endarterectomy, a procedure that continues to be performed today. Although his work was not published until 1959, carotid endarterectomy has since supplanted other surgical methods, providing excellent early and long-term results. It has become the most common surgical intervention in vascular surgery in all developed countries. In 1958, DeBakey also introduced bypass reconstruction of the supra-aortic branches into routine vascular surgery practice. He was a pioneering scientist, educator, and innovator.

Director, Methodist Heart & Vascular Center Houston [9]. DeBakey is one of the few surgeons who have graced the cover of Time magazine.

References

1. Min WD, Loftus CM. History of carotid surgery. Neurosurg Clin N Am. 2001;12:167–72.
2. Virchow R. Thrombose und Embolie. Gefassen Zundung und Septische Infektion. In: Gesammelte Abhandlungen zur Wissen Schaftlichen Medicin. Frankfurt: AM Meidinger; 1856. p. 219–732.
3. Chiari H. Ueber das Verhalten des teilungswinkels der carotis communis bei der endarteritis chronica deformans. Verh Dtsch Pathol GES. 1905;9:326–30.
4. Carrel A. The transplantation of organs: a preliminary communication. JAMA. 1905;45:1645–6.
5. Takayasu M. A case with peculiar cchanges of the central retinal vessels. Acta Soc Ophthalmol Japonicae, Tokyo. 1908;12:554.
6. Hunt JR. Hunt: the role of the carotid arteries: the role of the carotid arteries in the causation of vascular lesions of the brain, with remarks on certain special features of the symptomatology. 1914. Am J Med Sci. 2013;346(6):504–9.
7. Moniz E, Lima A, de Lacerda R. Hemiplegies par thorombose de la carotide interne. Presse Med. 1937;45:977–80.
8. Fisher M. Occlusion of the carotid arteries: further experiences. AMA Arch Neurol Psychiatry. 1954;72:187–204.
9. DeBakey ME. Successful carotid endarterectomy for cerebrovascular insufficiency. Nineteen-year follow-up. JAMA. 1975;233:1083–5.

Epidemiology and Pathology of Carotid Artery Diseases

3

Jes S. Lindholt

3.1 Atherosclerosis

3.1.1 Introduction

Carotid artery atherosclerosis is a common vascular disorder characterised by plaque deposition within the carotid arteries, major arteries supplying blood to the brain. Epidemiologically, it is associated with several risk factors and has significant implications for cardiovascular health.

3.1.2 Epidemiology of Carotid Artery Atherosclerosis

The prevalence of carotid artery atherosclerosis increases with age, with a higher incidence in older populations. Studies have shown that prevalence rates vary widely depending on the population studied and the diagnostic methods used.

For example, a meta-analysis by Song et al. (2017) estimated the prevalence of carotid artery atherosclerosis at around 30–40% in individuals aged 65 [1].

3.1.2.1 Risk Factors

1. Age: Aging is a significant risk factor for the development of carotid artery atherosclerosis, and plaque accumulation increases with age.
2. Gender: Men tend to have a higher prevalence of carotid artery atherosclerosis compared to premenopausal women. However, after menopause, the risk becomes similar between sexes.

J. S. Lindholt (✉)
Department of Cardiothoracic and Vascular Surgery, Odense University Hospital, Odense, Denmark
e-mail: jes.sanddal.lindholt@rsyd.dk

D. Radak, S. Duvnjak (eds.), *Carotid Artery Disease: Surgical Perspectives*, https://doi.org/10.1007/978-3-031-81842-4_3

3. Hypertension: High blood pressure is a significant risk factor associated with the development and progression of atherosclerosis.
4. Hyperlipidemia: Elevated levels of low-density lipoprotein (LDL) cholesterol and triglycerides contribute to plaque formation.
5. Diabetes mellitus: Both type 1 and type 2 diabetes are associated with an increased risk of atherosclerosis due to effects on vascular function and lipid metabolism.
6. Smoking: Tobacco use is a significant modifiable risk factor for atherosclerosis.
7. Obesity: Obesity, particularly central adiposity, is linked to a higher risk of atherosclerosis.
8. Family history: Genetic predisposition plays a role, and a family history of cardiovascular disease increases the risk.

3.1.2.2 Complications

Carotid artery atherosclerosis can lead to significant morbidity and mortality through embolic events or stenosis resulting in stroke. Atherosclerotic plaques in the carotid arteries may rupture, leading to thrombosis and subsequent cerebral ischemia [2].

3.1.2.3 Screening and Diagnosis

Imaging modalities such as carotid ultrasound, computed tomography angiography (CTA), and magnetic resonance angiography (MRA) are commonly used to diagnose and screen for carotid artery atherosclerosis. Carotid artery stenosis, measured as a percentage of luminal narrowing, is a critical diagnostic criterion [3].

3.1.3 Pathophysiology of Carotid Artery Atherosclerosis

Carotid atherosclerosis is characterised by plaque build-up in the carotid arteries, which supply blood to the brain, head, and neck. This build-up of plaque results from a complex interplay of various factors, including endothelial dysfunction, inflammation, lipid metabolism abnormalities, and vascular smooth muscle cell proliferation. Here's a breakdown of the pathophysiology:

1. Endothelial dysfunction: The endothelium, the inner lining of blood vessels, plays a crucial role in maintaining vascular health. Dysfunction can occur due to various factors, such as high blood pressure, smoking, diabetes, and high cholesterol levels. When the endothelium becomes damaged, it loses its ability to regulate vascular tone and permeability, making it more susceptible to accumulating lipids and inflammatory cells.
2. Formation of fatty streaks: Chronic endothelial dysfunction leads to low-density lipoprotein (LDL) cholesterol deposition within the arterial wall. These lipids accumulate in the subendothelial space, initiating the formation of fatty streaks, which are the earliest visible lesions of atherosclerosis.

3. Inflammation: LDL cholesterol within the arterial wall triggers an inflammatory response. Inflammatory cells, particularly monocytes and T lymphocytes, migrate into the vessel wall in response to chemokines and cytokines released by endothelial cells and other inflammatory cells. These immune cells become activated, producing inflammatory mediators such as cytokines, chemokines, and reactive oxygen species, further promoting the progression of atherosclerosis.
4. Foam cell formation: Monocytes that migrate into the arterial wall differentiate into macrophages. These macrophages engulf the oxidised LDL particles, transforming them into foam cells. Foam cells are a hallmark of early atherosclerotic lesions and contribute to forming fatty plaques.
5. Smooth muscle cell proliferation and fibrosis: In response to inflammatory signals and growth factors released by activated macrophages and endothelial cells, vascular smooth muscle cells migrate from the media to the intima of the artery and proliferate. Smooth muscle cells contribute to forming a fibrous cap over the fatty plaque. However, excessive smooth muscle cell proliferation can lead to plaque instability and rupture.
6. Plaque formation and progression: Over time, the accumulation of lipids, inflammatory cells, and smooth muscle cells leads to atherosclerotic plaques. These plaques may protrude into the arterial lumen, causing narrowing and potentially reducing blood flow to the brain. Plaque rupture or erosion can trigger thrombus formation, leading to acute thrombotic events such as stroke or transient ischemic attack (TIA) [4, 5].

3.2 Arterial Dissection

3.2.1 Introduction

Carotid artery dissection is a condition that occurs when the layers of the carotid artery wall tear, leading to blood flow between the layers and potentially causing stroke or transient ischemic attack (TIA).

3.2.2 Epidemiology of Carotid Artery Dissection

Carotid artery dissection is a relatively rare condition, but it is a significant cause of stroke, particularly in young and middle-aged adults. The annual incidence of spontaneous carotid artery dissection is estimated to be between 2.5 and 3 per 100,000 people [6]. Traumatic carotid artery dissection is more common in younger individuals, often resulting from blunt or penetrating neck trauma.

Age and gender distribution: While carotid artery dissection can occur at any age, it most commonly affects individuals between the ages of 30 and 50 years old. There appears to be a slight male predominance in spontaneous carotid artery dissection cases, with some studies reporting a male-to-female ratio of approximately 3:2 [7].

3.2.2.1 Risk Factors

1. Trauma: Trauma is a significant risk factor for carotid artery dissection. This can include motor vehicle accidents, sports injuries, falls, and even minor trauma such as chiropractic manipulation or vigorous neck movements.
2. Connective tissue disorders: Certain connective tissue disorders, such as Ehlers-Danlos syndrome and Marfan syndrome, increase the risk of arterial dissections due to inherent weakness in the vessel walls.
3. Genetic factors: Genetic predispositions may increase susceptibility to carotid artery dissection.
4. Other conditions: Fibromuscular dysplasia, arterial tortuosity, and atherosclerosis may also predispose individuals to carotid artery dissection.

3.2.2.2 Clinical Presentation

Symptoms of carotid artery dissection can include unilateral headache, neck pain, Horner syndrome (ptosis, miosis, and anhidrosis), pulsatile tinnitus, and signs of cerebral or retinal ischemia such as visual disturbances, weakness, or speech difficulties.

3.2.2.3 Diagnosis

Diagnosis is often made through imaging studies such as magnetic resonance angiography (MRA), computed tomography angiography (CTA), or Doppler ultrasound.

Digital subtraction angiography (DSA) remains the gold standard for diagnosis but is usually reserved for cases where non-invasive imaging is inconclusive or further characterisation is needed.

3.2.2.4 Treatment

Treatment may include anticoagulation or antiplatelet therapy to prevent thromboembolic complications. In some cases, endovascular interventions such as stenting or angioplasty may be necessary to restore blood flow in the affected artery. Surgery may also be indicated in some instances, mainly if there is evidence of ongoing ischemia or if the dissection is causing significant neurological symptoms.

3.2.3 Pathophysiology of Carotid Artery Dissection

1. Initiation of dissection: Carotid artery dissections can be spontaneous or traumatic. Spontaneous dissections often occur due to underlying connective tissue disorders, such as Ehlers-Danlos syndrome or Marfan syndrome. In contrast, traumatic dissections result from sudden movements or blunt force trauma to the neck.
2. Tear formation: Tears typically occur in the innermost layer of the arterial wall, the intima. Blood then enters the tear, causing the layers of the arterial wall to separate.
3. Formation of false lumen: As blood enters the tear, it creates a false lumen between the layers of the arterial wall. This false lumen can extend along the

length of the artery and lead to the compression of the true lumen, reducing blood flow.
4. Thrombus formation: Blood within the false lumen can stagnate, forming a thrombus or blood clot. This thrombus can further occlude the artery, leading to ischemia or embolisation.
5. Hematoma formation: Blood may also accumulate within the arterial wall, forming a hematoma. This can further compress the true lumen and compromise blood flow.
6. Ischemia and neurological deficits: Reduced blood flow through the carotid artery can lead to ischemia in the brain, resulting in neurological deficits such as transient ischemic attacks (TIAs) or ischemic strokes [7, 8].

It's worth noting that the pathophysiology of carotid artery dissections can vary depending on factors such as the underlying cause, the extent of the tear, and the presence of additional risk factors [9].

3.3 Aneurysm

3.3.1 Introduction

Carotid artery aneurysms are relatively rare but potentially severe vascular abnormalities.

3.3.2 Epidemiology of Carotid Artery Aneurysm

Carotid artery aneurysms are less common than aneurysms in other arterial locations, such as the aorta or cerebral arteries. The incidence of carotid artery aneurysms is estimated to be between 0.4% and 4% of all peripheral artery aneurysms. They occur more frequently in older age groups, with the average age of diagnosis ranging from 60 to 70 years. Some studies have a slight male predominance, affecting males more frequently than females [10].

3.3.2.1 Etiology and Risk Factors

Atherosclerosis is the most common cause of carotid artery aneurysms, particularly in elderly patients. Other causes include trauma, connective tissue disorders (such as Ehlers-Danlos syndrome and Marfan syndrome), infection (e.g. syphilis), and iatrogenic injury. Risk factors for carotid artery aneurysms include hypertension, smoking, hyperlipidemia, and a family history of vascular diseases.

3.3.2.2 Clinical Presentation

Carotid artery aneurysms are often asymptomatic and may be incidentally discovered during imaging studies for unrelated conditions. Symptoms may arise due to compression of adjacent structures or embolisation of thrombus or plaque from the aneurysm. Common symptoms include neck mass, pulsatile mass, neurological deficits (such as transient ischemic attacks or strokes), and cranial nerve palsies [11].

3.3.2.3 Diagnosis

Diagnosis is typically confirmed through imaging studies such as ultrasound, computed tomography angiography (CTA), magnetic resonance angiography (MRA), or conventional angiography. Imaging helps determine the aneurysm's size, location, and morphology and identify any associated thrombus or embolic complications.

3.3.2.4 Treatment

Treatment options depend on various factors, including the size and location of the aneurysm, the presence of symptoms, and the patient's overall health. Small, asymptomatic aneurysms may be managed conservatively with close monitoring. Surgical interventions, such as aneurysm resection with or without bypass grafting, may be required for symptomatic or enlarging aneurysms to prevent complications such as rupture or embolisation [12].

3.3.3 Pathophysiology of Carotid Artery Aneurysm

A carotid aneurysm is an abnormal dilation or bulging in the wall of the carotid artery. It can occur in the common carotid artery, internal carotid artery, or external carotid artery. The pathophysiology of carotid aneurysm involves various factors, including hemodynamic stress, atherosclerosis, genetic predisposition, and inflammatory processes [13].

1. Hemodynamic stress: High blood pressure and turbulent blood flow can weaken the arterial wall over time, leading to the formation of aneurysms. Areas of the artery exposed to increased stress, such as bifurcations or curves, are particularly susceptible.
2. Atherosclerosis: Atherosclerosis significantly contributes to the development of carotid aneurysms. It involves the build-up of plaque on the inner walls of arteries. Over time, plaque accumulation can weaken the arterial wall and contribute to aneurysm formation.
3. Genetic predisposition: Genetic factors can play a role in the development of carotid aneurysms. Certain genetic conditions, such as connective tissue disorders like Marfan syndrome and Ehlers-Danlos syndrome, predispose individuals to arterial weakness and aneurysm formation.
4. Inflammatory processes: Chronic inflammation within the arterial wall can weaken the tissue and contribute to aneurysm formation. Inflammatory conditions such as vasculitis or infections may weaken the arterial wall and subsequent aneurysm development.
5. Trauma: Traumatic injury to the carotid artery can cause focal weakness or damage to the arterial wall, increasing the risk of aneurysm formation.

6. Congenital abnormalities: Rarely, congenital abnormalities in the structure of the carotid artery can predispose individuals to aneurysm formation [14, 15].

The exact mechanisms underlying carotid aneurysm formation may vary depending on the individual and the underlying causes. However, the common theme involves the weakening of the arterial wall, which leads to its dilation and eventual aneurysm formation.

3.4 Vasculitis

3.4.1 Introduction

Carotid vasculitis is a rare condition characterised by inflammation of the carotid arteries, which are major blood vessels supplying the head and neck. If not promptly diagnosed and treated, it can lead to significant morbidity and mortality.

3.4.2 Epidemiology of Carotid Artery Vasculitis

Rare disease: Carotid vasculitis is considered a rare disease, with limited epidemiological data available.

Age and gender: It can affect individuals of any age but is more commonly seen in adults, particularly those in their 40s to 60s. There seems to be a slight male predominance, although this is not consistently reported across studies [16].

3.4.2.1 Etiology and Risk Factors

Autoimmune disorders: Carotid vasculitis is often associated with autoimmune diseases such as rheumatoid arthritis, systemic lupus erythematosus (SLE), giant cell arteritis, and Takayasu arteritis. These conditions can trigger inflammation within the blood vessels, leading to vasculitis.

Infections: Certain infections, including bacterial and viral infections, have been implicated in the pathogenesis of vasculitis although the exact mechanisms are not fully understood.

Environmental factors: Environmental factors, such as exposure to toxins or pollutants, may contribute to the development of vasculitis, but this requires further investigation.

3.4.2.2 Clinical Presentation

Symptoms: The clinical presentation of carotid vasculitis can vary widely depending on the extent and severity of arterial involvement. Common symptoms include headache, neck pain, visual disturbances, transient ischemic attacks (TIAs), and stroke.

Complications: If left untreated, carotid vasculitis can lead to severe complications such as ischemic stroke, carotid artery dissection, and aneurysm formation.

3.4.2.3 Diagnosis

Imaging: Diagnosis is typically made through imaging studies such as Doppler ultrasound, CT angiography (CTA), magnetic resonance angiography (MRA), or conventional angiography. These tests can reveal arterial wall thickening, stenosis, or aneurysmal changes indicative of vasculitis.

Biopsy: In some cases, a biopsy of the affected artery may be necessary to confirm the diagnosis. However, this is less commonly performed due to the risks associated with invasive procedures.

3.4.2.4 Treatment and Prognosis

Immunosuppressive therapy: Treatment usually involves immunosuppressive medications such as corticosteroids, methotrexate, or other disease-modifying antirheumatic drugs (DMARDs) to suppress the inflammatory response and prevent further damage to the arteries [17, 18].

Anticoagulation: Anticoagulation therapy may be necessary for thrombosis or embolism associated with carotid vasculitis.

Prognosis: The prognosis varies depending on the underlying cause, extent of arterial involvement, and treatment response. Early diagnosis and aggressive management are crucial to improve outcomes and reduce the risk of complications.

3.4.3 Pathophysiology of Carotid Artery Vasculitis

Carotid vasculitis is a rare condition characterised by inflammation of the carotid artery. It can lead to a range of symptoms, including headaches, transient ischemic attacks (TIAs), stroke, and, in severe cases, carotid artery stenosis or occlusion.

While the exact cause of carotid vasculitis is not always clear, it is often associated with autoimmune disorders such as giant cell arteritis, Takayasu arteritis, or systemic lupus erythematosus (SLE), though it can also occur idiopathically.

3.4.3.1 Pathophysiology

1. Immune dysregulation:

   In autoimmune conditions like giant cell arteritis or Takayasu arteritis, the immune system mistakenly attacks the arterial wall, leading to inflammation. This immune response involves T lymphocytes, macrophages, and other inflammatory cells infiltrating the arterial wall.
2. Vascular damage:

   The inflammatory process causes damage to the endothelial lining of the artery, disrupting its normal function. This damage triggers further inflammatory responses and can lead to the formation of plaques or narrowing of the artery.
3. Thrombosis and ischemia:

   Inflammation and damage to the arterial wall can promote the formation of blood clots (thrombosis). Thrombosis may result in partial or complete blockage of the carotid artery, leading to reduced blood flow to the brain. Depending on the severity and duration of the blockage, reduced blood flow can cause transient ischemic attacks (TIAs) or strokes.

4. Fibrosis and stenosis:

   Chronic inflammation can lead to collagen and fibrous tissue deposition in the arterial wall. This fibrosis can cause the carotid artery to narrow (stenosis), further compromising blood flow to the brain. Severe stenosis increases the risk of stroke.

5. Rupture and aneurysm formation:

   In advanced cases, chronic inflammation weakens the arterial wall, increasing the risk of rupture. Rupture of the carotid artery can lead to bleeding and stroke. Additionally, aneurysms may develop due to the weakening of the arterial wall [19–21].

References

1. Song P, Fang Z, Wang H, et al. Global prevalence of atherosclerotic cardiovascular disease in people with atherosclerotic cardiovascular disease: protocol for a systematic review and meta-analysis. JMIR Res Protoc. 2017;6(6):e127. https://doi.org/10.2196/resprot.7798.
2. Weber C, Noels H. Atherosclerosis: current pathogenesis and therapeutic options. Nat Med. 2011;17(11):1410–22. https://doi.org/10.1038/nm.2538.
3. Goldstein LB, Bushnell CD, Adams RJ, et al. Guidelines for the primary prevention of stroke. Stroke. 2011;42(2):517–84. https://doi.org/10.1161/STR.0b013e3181fcb238.
4. Ross R. Atherosclerosis—an inflammatory disease. N Engl J Med. 1999;340(2):115–26.
5. Libby P, Ridker PM, Hansson GK. Progress and challenges in translating the biology of atherosclerosis. Nature. 2011;473(7347):317–25.
6. Lee VH, Brown RD Jr, Mandrekar JN, Mokri B. Incidence and outcome of cervical artery dissection: a population-based study. Neurology. 2006;67(10):1809–12.
7. Debette S, Leys D. Cervical-artery dissections: predisposing factors, diagnosis, and outcome. Lancet Neurol. 2009;8(7):668–78.
8. Arnold M, Bousser MG, Fahrni G. Carotid dissection. Neurol Clin. 2006;24(1):49–57.
9. Lyrer PA, Engelter ST. Antithrombotic drugs for carotid artery dissection. Stroke. 2010;41(3):e85.
10. Gupta V, Nwobi O, Asmarats L, et al. Epidemiology, pathophysiology, and natural history of aortic aneurysms. In: StatPearls [Internet]. Treasure Island: StatPearls Publishing; 2022.
11. McCready RA, Bryant MA, Divelbiss JL, et al. Carotid artery aneurysms: a case report and review of the literature. J Vasc Surg. 2007;45(1):154–60. https://doi.org/10.1016/j.jvs.2006.09.036.
12. Chaloupka JC, Putman CM, Citardi MJ, et al. Endovascular therapy for giant aneurysms of the carotid circulation. Neurosurgery. 1999;44(4):713–21. https://doi.org/10.1097/00006123-199904000-00038.
13. Rangel-Castilla L, Kalani MY, Sweeney JM, et al. Pathogenesis, diagnosis, and management of carotid artery aneurysms and pseudoaneurysms. Neurosurg Focus. 2011;30(6):E11.
14. Muneer K, Singla A, Jain A, Bhatnagar A, Vashishtha RK. A review of carotid artery aneurysms: from etiopathogenesis to management. Cureus. 2019;11(8):e5406.
15. Kadirvel R, Ding YH, Dai D, Rezek I, Lewis DA, Kallmes DF. The influence of hemodynamic forces on biomarkers in rabbits' walls of elastase-induced aneurysms. Neuroradiology. 2007;49(12):1041–53.
16. Jennette JC, Falk RJ, Bacon PA, et al. 2012 revised International Chapel Hill Consensus Conference Nomenclature of Vasculitides. Arthritis Rheum. 2013;65(1):1–11.

17. Salvarani C, Brown RD Jr, Calamia KT, et al. Primary central nervous system vasculitis: analysis of 101 patients. Ann Neurol. 2007;62(5):442–51.
18. García-Martínez A, Hernández-Rodríguez J, Espígol-Frigolé G, et al. Clinical relevance of persistently elevated circulating cytokines (tumor necrosis factor ? and interleukin-6) in the long-term follow-up of patients with giant cell arteritis. Arthritis Care Res (Hoboken). 2010;62(6):835–41.
19. Salvarani C, Cantini F, Hunder GG. Polymyalgia rheumatica and giant-cell arteritis. Lancet. 2008;372(9634):234–45. https://doi.org/10.1016/S0140-6736(08)61077-9.
20. Johnston SL, Lock RJ, Gompels MM. Takayasu arteritis: a review. J Clin Pathol. 2002;55(7):481–6. https://doi.org/10.1136/jcp.55.7.481.
21. Watanabe R, Ishii T, Nakamura K, et al. Vascular lesions in systemic lupus erythematosus. Autoimmun Rev. 2010;9(4):259–64. https://doi.org/10.1016/j.autrev.2009.10.003.

Diagnosis of Carotid Artery Diseases

4

Stevo Duvnjak and Djordje Radak

The diagnosis of carotid artery disease includes:
- Vascular examination
- Focused neurological examination
- Color duplex ultrasonography of the carotid and vertebral arteries
- Computed tomography (CT) or magnetic resonance angiography (MRI) of the aortic arch, carotid arteries, vertebral arteries, and intracranial vessels

4.1 Clinical Vascular Examination

4.1.1 Introduction

The symptomatic stage of the carotid disease is manifested by a transient or permanent neurological deficit in the anterior (carotid) or posterior (vertebral) segment. Carotid atherosclerotic disease is the cause of about 70% of cases of cerebral ischemia [1]. TOAST trial classified five different subtypes of ischemic stroke: (1) strokes due to cardioembolic events (27%); (2) cryptogenic strokes (35%); (3) strokes from large-artery atherosclerosis (13%); (4) strokes due to small-vessel disease (23%); and (5) strokes of other determined etiology (2% of cases) [2]. The most important thing is that this segment is available for successful, fast, and

S. Duvnjak (✉)
Department of Vascular Surgery, Rigshospitalet, Copenhagen, Denmark
e-mail: stevo.duvnjak@regionh.dk

D. Radak
Serbian Academy of Sciences and Arts, Belgrade, Serbia

Clinic for Surgery, Euromedik Hospital, Belgrade, Serbia
e-mail: radak@ikvbd.com

D. Radak, S. Duvnjak (eds.), *Carotid Artery Disease: Surgical Perspectives*,
https://doi.org/10.1007/978-3-031-81842-4_4

effective revascularization interventions. Early diagnosis and treatment are essential to avoid further complications of insufficient brain nutrition. Most often, all the manifestations of a stroke develop to their full extent within a few minutes to about a couple of hours. Typical is the appearance of weakness or loss of one half of the body, numbness of one half of the face and body, difficulties in speaking or understanding speech such as dysphasia, loss of vision in one half of the visual field, loss of coordination of limb movements on one side, or sudden loss of balance and difficulty in walking [3].

According to the National Institute of Health Stroke Scale (NIHSS) [4] and the severity and frequency of brain ischemia symptoms, we can distinguish:

1. **Transient ischemic attack (TIA): focal ischemic neurological deficit that lasts a few minutes to 24 h, resolves without consequences, but tends to recur.**
2. **Single TIA: complete resolution of neurological symptoms during 24 h.**
3. **Crescendo TIA: multiple episodes with neurological deficit, which last from a few minutes to over 24 h, but with complete resolution of the neurological deficit between attacks.**
4. **Stroke in evolution: progression of the symptoms and neurological deficit over days without resolution of symptoms.**
5. **Minor stroke: neurological deficit lasting over 24 h but recovery without residual impairment.**
6. **Major non-disabling stroke: neurological deficit lasting over 24 h with residual impairment.**

4.1.2 Physical Examination

A vascular examination begins with a detailed medical history, including the patient's description of neurological symptoms, such as the onset, character, recurrence, and duration. Patients with carotid stenosis can also be asymptomatic. Additionally, other relevant conditions, such as heart disease (particularly rhythm disorders), peripheral vascular disease, and aneurysms, should be noted. Prior surgeries, especially neck surgery, may necessitate further examination of the vocal cords to prevent severe complications during carotid surgery. Risk factors such as obesity, hypertension, diabetes mellitus, smoking, high lipid levels, and physical inactivity should also be recorded. All medications, particularly antiplatelet agents, lipid-lowering drugs, and antihypertensive drugs, must be noted.

The physical examination begins with blood pressure measurement in both arms and pulse examination, typically of the brachial and radial arteries, assessing the rhythm and quality of the pulses (Fig. 4.1). Key areas for carotid vascular examination, palpation, and auscultation include the mandibular angle and supraclavicular region (Fig. 4.2). Any bruits may indicate carotid artery stenosis, warranting further examination with ultrasound.

The vascular examination continues with the palpation of the abdominal aorta to check for a potential aneurysm (Fig. 4.3). Additionally, the femoral, popliteal, and pedal arteries are examined through pulse palpation (Fig. 4.4).

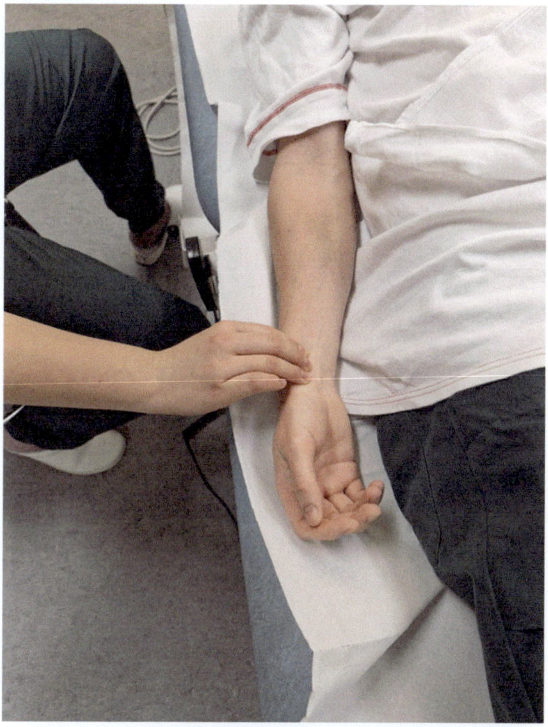

Fig. 4.1 The radial pulse is weakened in the case of stenosis of the arteries of the proximal segment and absent if they are entirely closed

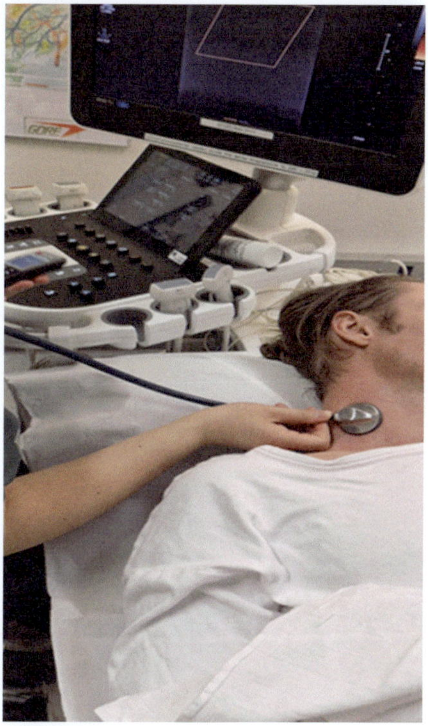

Fig. 4.2 Typical examination sites for carotid artery palpation and auscultation

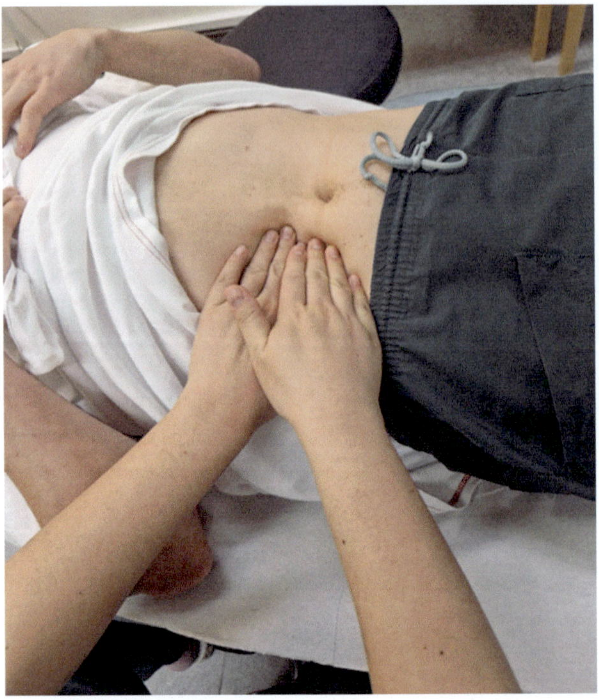

Fig. 4.3 Palpation of the abdominal aorta should always be performed during a vascular examination, as it can help detect potential aneurysmal disease

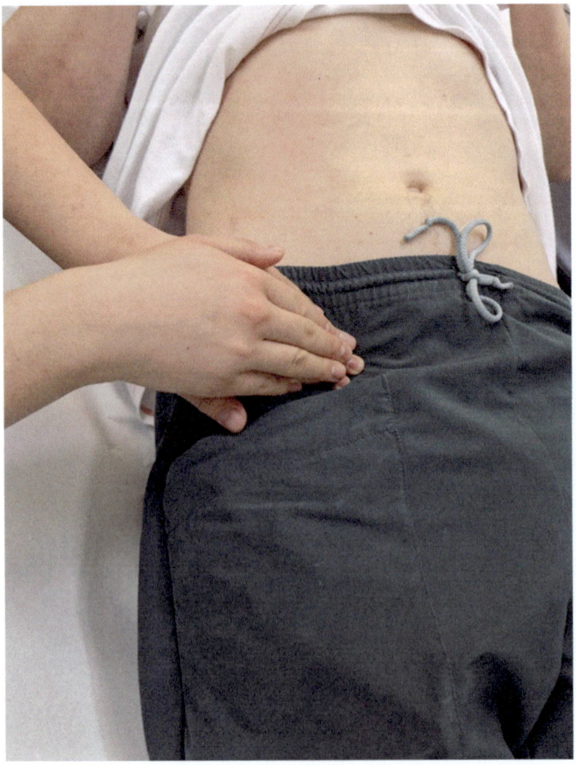

Fig. 4.4 Palpation of the femoral arteries can help detect potential aneurysmal or occlusive disease

4.2 Vascular Surgery Focused Neurological Examination

4.2.1 Introduction

Focal ischemia of the brain most commonly occurs due to embolization from an atherosclerotic plaque or atrial fibrillation affecting a specific cerebral artery. Other causes, such as a mobile thrombus in the ascending aorta and aortic arch, carotid dissection, aneurysm, and vasculitis, are less common causes of cerebral ischemia. Symptoms depend on the location and extent of arterial occlusion. A neurological examination can anatomically locate which brain area is ischemic based on the symptoms.

Symptoms and signs of ischemia in the carotid vascular region include amaurosis fugax (ipsilateral blindness), hemiparesis, hemiplegia, aphasia, and dysphasia. Symptoms and signs of vertebrobasilar insufficiency include dizziness, vomiting, nystagmus, diplopia, ataxia, bilateral motor or sensory deficits, unsteadiness when walking, homonymous visual defects, dysarthria, and drop attacks (sudden falls without loss of consciousness).

The modified Rankin Scale (mRS) is commonly used to determine indications for surgical treatment. According to guidelines, symptomatic patients with an mRS score of less than 3 are candidates for surgery. Patients with an mRS score greater than 3 should be reevaluated for surgery after rehabilitation [1].

Modified Rankin Scale—mRS [5]

0 point—No symptoms

1-point—Able to perform all usual duties and activities (no significant disability)

2-points—Unable to perform all previous activities but able to look after own affairs without assistance (slight disability)

3-points—Requires some help, but able to walk without assistance (moderate disability)

4-points—Unable to walk without assistance and unable to attend to own bodily needs without assistance (moderately severe disability)

5-points—Incontinent and requires constant nursing care and attention (severe disability)

6-points—Death

4.2.2 Cranial and Peripheral Nerve Examination

Focused vascular surgery neurological examination includes cranial and peripheral nerve examination [6, 7].

4.2.2.1 Cranial Nerve Examination

Olfactory Nerve (I) (Smell Function): Ask the patient if they have noticed any changes in their sense of smell.

Optic Nerve (II): Assess standard visual fields for both binocular and monocular vision without ophthalmoscopic examination.

Oculomotor Nerve (III): Check for normal pupillary light reactions, appropriate pupil size, and normal eyeball movement.

Trochlear Nerve (IV): Evaluate for downward and lateral eyeball movement.

Trigeminal Nerve (V): Test for normal sensation in all three branches (ophthalmic, maxillary, and mandibular) with light touch.

Abducens Nerve (VI): Assess for lateral eye movements.

Facial Nerve (VII): Check for normal and equal strength during facial movements such as frowning, squinting, showing teeth, and puffing cheeks. The taste sensation on the anterior part of the tongue is not examined.

Vestibulocochlear Nerve (VIII): Test for normal hearing by using finger rubbing.

Glossopharyngeal Nerve (IX): Ensure no difficulty in swallowing, a normal gag reflex, and normal taste sensation.

Vagus Nerve (X): Check for a normal voice with no hoarseness and no deviation of the palate or uvula.

Accessory Nerve (XI): Evaluate shoulder shrug and head turning against resistance.

Hypoglossal Nerve (XII): Ensure no tongue deviation.

4.2.2.2 Peripheral Nerve Examination

Extremities Motor Function: Normal and equal muscle tone in both upper and lower extremities, without spasticity or clonus. Normal and equal strength in the shoulders, hips, knees, and ankles. Normal dorsal and palmar flexion of the wrists. Extended arm test shows no pronation or downward drift.

Extremity Sensibility: Normal and equal sensation in both upper and lower extremities upon light touch.

Coordination: Normal Stewart-Holmes test, Romberg test, diadochokinesia test, and arm and leg roll test, with no asymmetry.

Walk: Normal walk, including walking on heels and toes. Line walking shows no balance disturbance.

4.3 Ultrasound of Carotid Artery

4.3.1 Introduction

Color duplex ultrasonography (CDU) is a completely noninvasive, simple, cost-effective, rapid, and reliable method for diagnosing extracranial arteries supplying the brain. CDU allows for the assessment of stenosis severity, morphological characteristics of plaques (such as echogenicity), and the hemodynamic significance of stenosis using B-mode imaging, color flow Doppler, and spectral analysis.

Spectral analysis is a crucial component of the examination, providing information on whether arterial narrowing has led to significant stenosis and reduced blood flow.

For diagnosing carotid stenosis greater than 70%, a peak systolic velocity greater than 200 cm/s has a sensitivity of 90% and a specificity of 94%. For diagnosing carotid stenosis greater than 50%, the specificity is slightly lower at 88%, but the sensitivity remains high at 98% when using a peak systolic velocity threshold of greater than 150 cm/s as a threshold value [8, 9].

4.3.2 B-Mode Ultrasound Examination

B-mode, or grayscale mode, is used to initiate the carotid examination in both longitudinal and transverse views to localize the carotid vessels and bifurcation (Fig. 4.5). The patient can be positioned differently for the examination, (Fig. 4.6) typically showing the common positioning during the procedure. B-mode imaging provides information on carotid plaque echogenicity, which can be classified as hypoechogenic, isoechogenic, or hyperechogenic. Additionally, B-mode can reveal plaque irregularity and possible ulceration, which are considered features of complicated plaque.

B-mode imaging alone cannot provide precise measurements of lumen size and blood flow. However, when combined with color Doppler and spectral analysis, it offers comprehensive information. Hyperechogenic plaques, such as those with calcifications, can present challenges during the examination due to shadowing effects. In such cases, assessing color flow and spectral analysis both distal and proximal to the plaque helps determine the degree of stenosis (Fig. 4.7).

Isoechogenic plaques are generally considered more stable (Fig. 4.8), whereas hypoechogenic plaques are often regarded as unstable and have a higher potential for complications (Fig. 4.9).

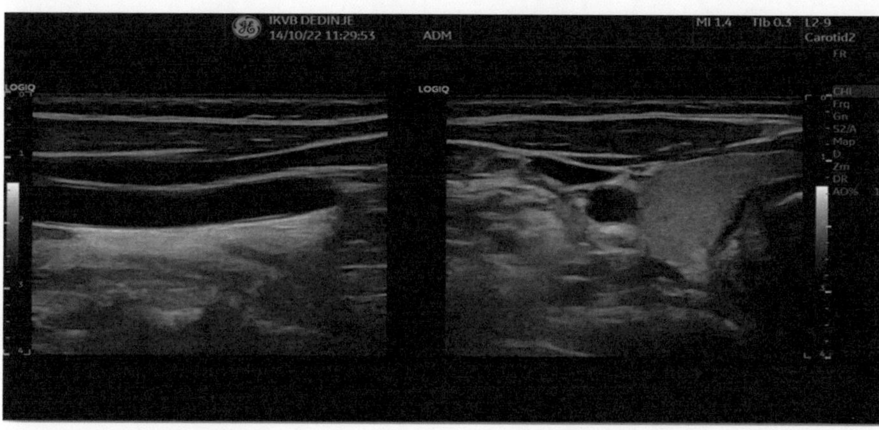

Fig. 4.5 B-mode imaging in longitudinal and transverse views of a normal carotid artery

Fig. 4.6 The patient is positioned appropriately, and a linear transducer with a frequency of 5–10 MHz is typically used for both longitudinal and transverse carotid artery scans

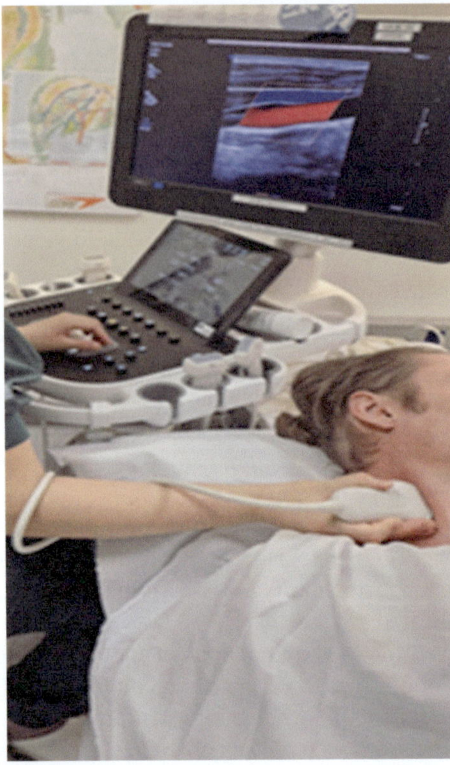

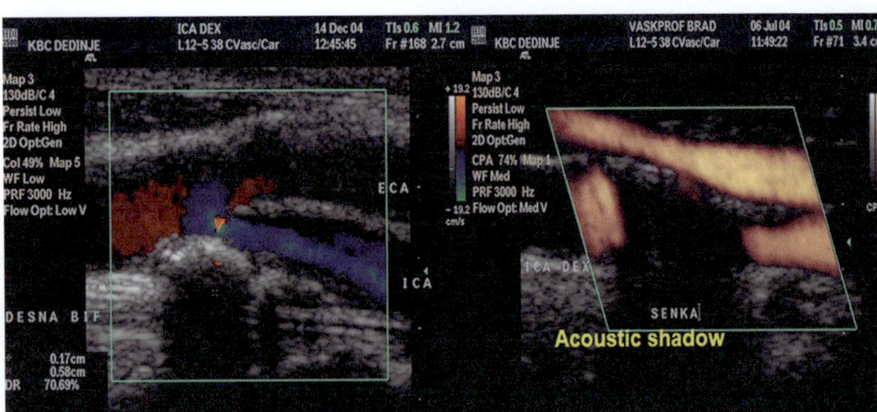

Fig. 4.7 Calcified carotid plaque with acoustic shadowing

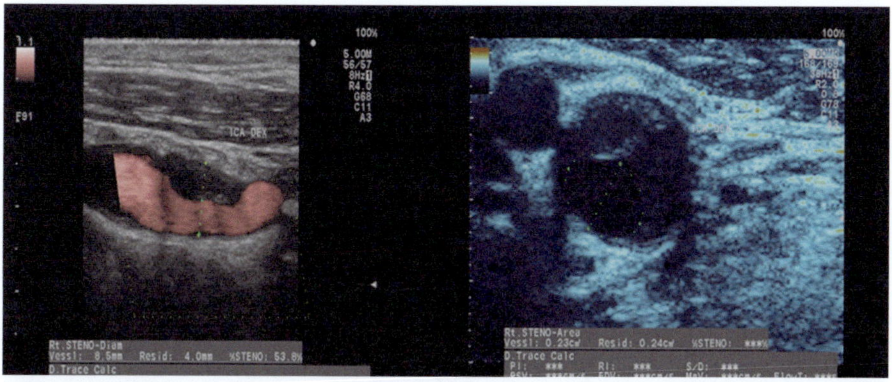

Fig. 4.8 Isoechogenic plaque in the internal carotid artery

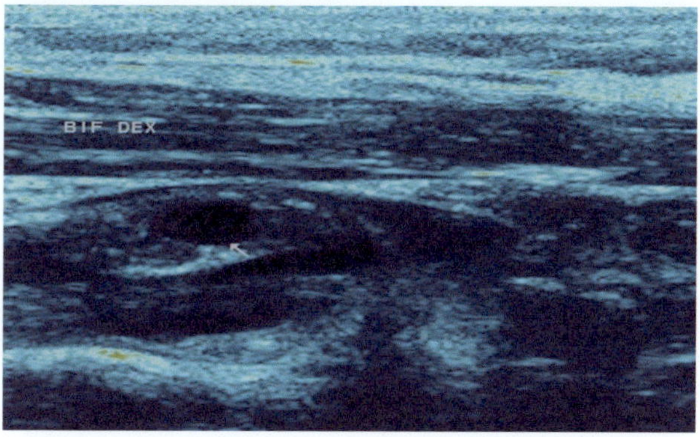

Fig. 4.9 Hypoechogenic plaque in the carotid artery with intraplaque hemorrhage has a higher embolic potential

4.3.3 Spectral Analysis

Spectral analysis is an integral part of ultrasound examination for arteries, enabling the assessment of flow quality and stenosis severity. A normal arterial vessel typically exhibits a triphasic waveform, indicating preserved flow and elasticity (Fig. 4.10). In cases of stenosis, higher peak systolic velocity (PSV) is recorded at the site of narrowing, which is proportional to the degree of stenosis. Key parameters for assessing stenosis include PSV, end-diastolic velocity (EDV), and the PSV ratio between the internal and common carotid arteries (Fig. 4.11).

In clinical practice, carotid stenosis is categorized as follows:

- **<50% stenosis:** No treatment required.
- **50–69% stenosis:** PSV of 125–230 cm/s; EDV of 100 cm/s; PSV ratio >2. Symptomatic patients may require treatment.
- **>70% stenosis:** PSV >230 cm/s; EDV >100 cm/s; PSV ratio >4. Symptomatic patients require treatment (Fig. 4.12).

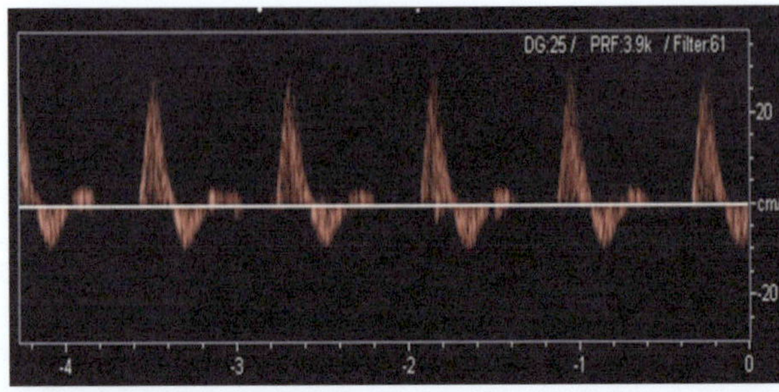

Fig. 4.10 Triphasic waveform in a normal artery during spectral analysis

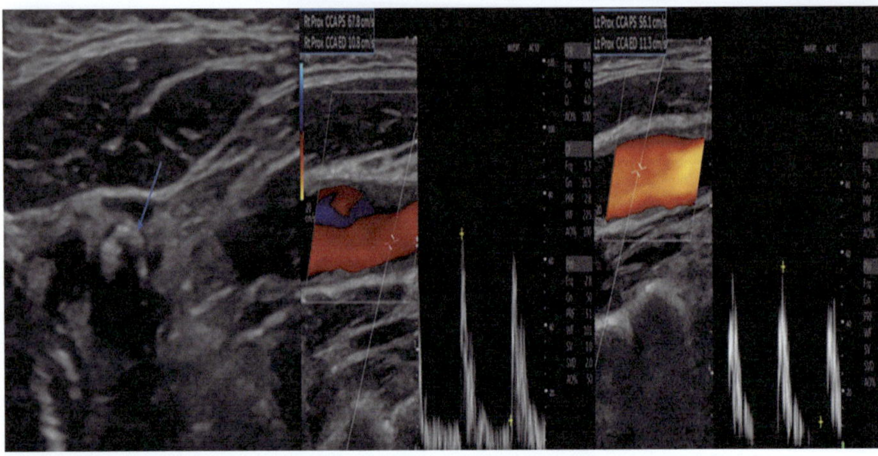

Fig. 4.11 B-mode imaging, color flow Doppler, and spectral analysis with Doppler angulation of less than 60 degrees reveal calcified plaque with a peak systolic velocity (PSV) greater than 230 cm/s, indicating significant stenosis in the internal carotid artery

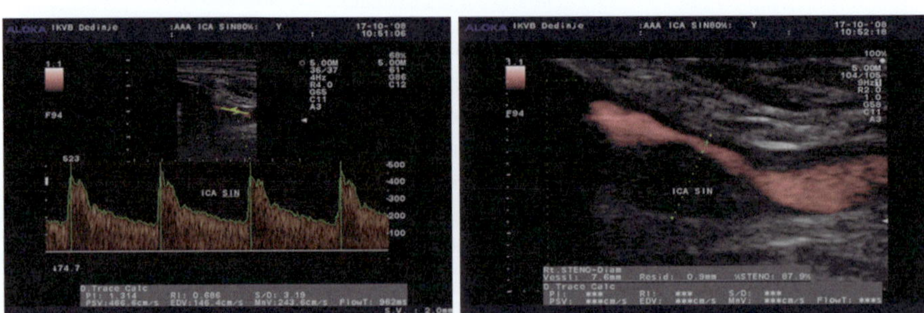

Fig. 4.12 A peak systolic velocity (PSV) greater than 230 cm/s indicates significant stenosis of the internal carotid artery. Power Doppler mode further confirms the presence of significant stenosis

Additionally, there are specific categories for patients with occluded internal carotid arteries (Fig. 4.13) and near occlusion (Fig. 4.14).

A vascular surgeon is interested in evaluating the morphology of the carotid plaque and the degree of stenosis.

When determining the indication for treatment, in addition to the degree of stenosis, essential parameters include the length of the stenosis, the configuration and echogenic characteristics of the plaque (e.g., fibrous, calcified, or with intraplaque hemorrhage), and the accessibility of the distal internal carotid artery for surgery. An ulcerated carotid plaque often causes symptoms such as transient ischemic

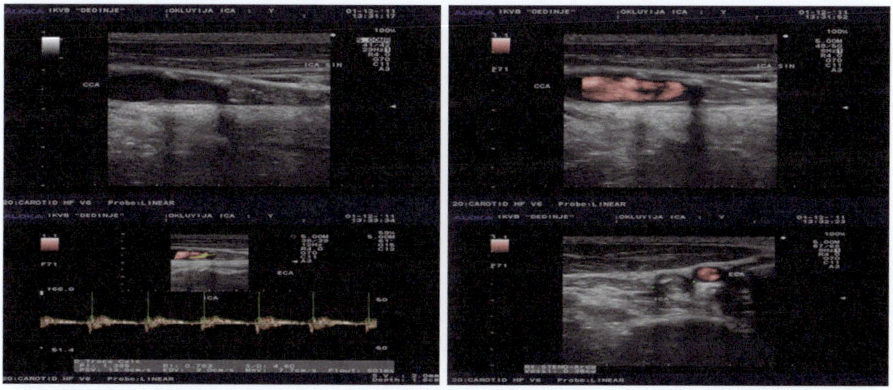

Fig. 4.13 Occlusion of the internal carotid artery is indicated by B-mode imaging and power Doppler mode showing no flow in the internal carotid artery. Spectral analysis may reveal a pre-occlusive Doppler spectral signal in the common carotid artery

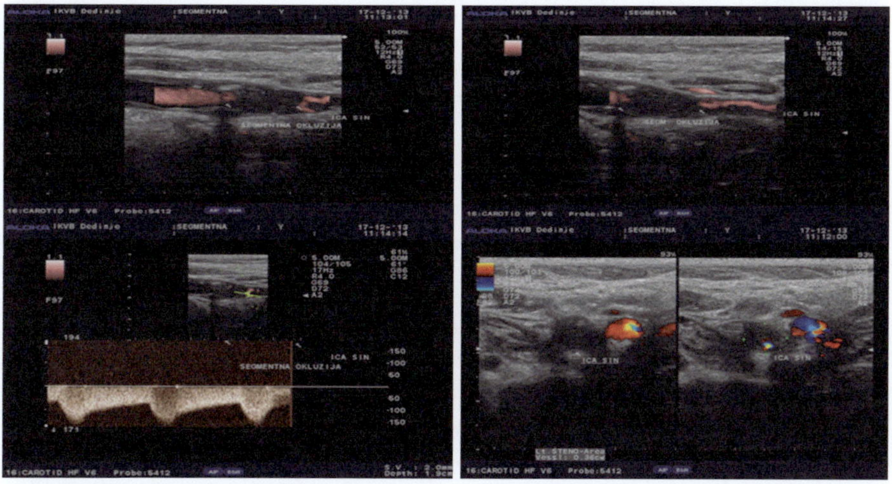

Fig. 4.14 Internal carotid artery occlusion with retrograde flow from the contralateral side observed in the distal segment of the ipsilateral internal carotid artery

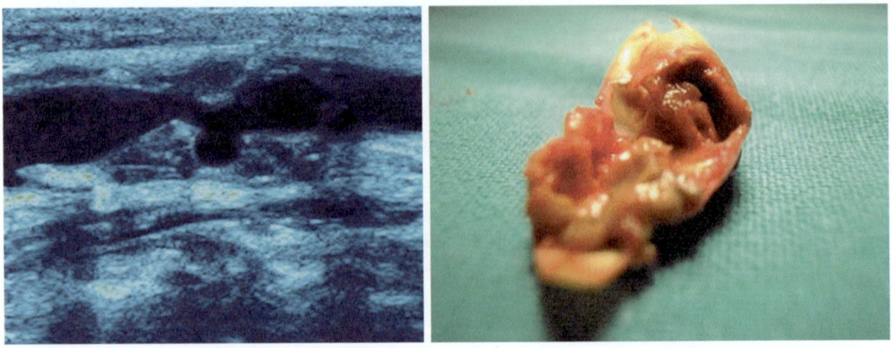

Fig. 4.15 Symptomatic subocclusion with a crescent TIA and ulcerated necrotic plaque was identified. An urgent carotid endarterectomy was performed

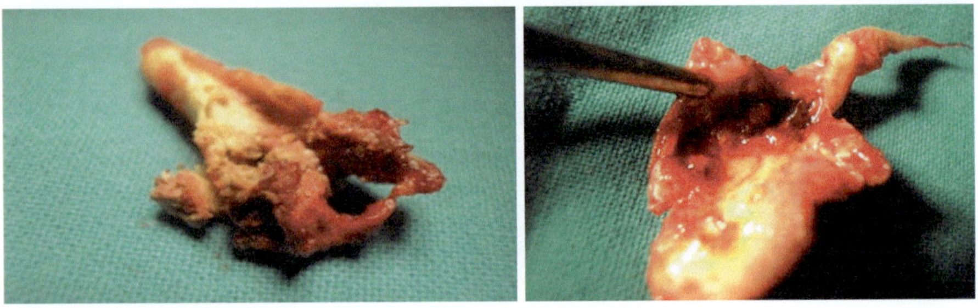

Fig. 4.16 A heterogeneous plaque with adjacent thrombosis is prone to embolization and may present with multiple episodes of transient ischemic attacks (TIAs)

attacks (TIAs) or strokes, highlighting the need for surgical intervention. Patients presenting with acute symptoms of cerebral ischemia typically have unstable or vulnerable plaques, frequently associated with floating thrombi that pose a risk of causing a more severe ischemic event (Figs. 4.15 and 4.16).

4.3.4 Color Flow Analysis

Blood flow through the arteries is typically laminar and forward during the cardiac cycle. Color flow ultrasonography allows for the examination of flow direction and velocity and helps to localize plaques and stenoses, which facilitates precise subsequent spectral analysis (Fig. 4.17). There are two modalities: color Doppler and power Doppler. The latter is independent of flow velocity and direction and can detect slower flow velocities (Figs. 4.18, 4.19, and 4.20).

Transcranial Doppler sonography, while not routinely used in extracranial carotid artery diseases, spectral wave analysis can indirectly provide information about flow direction, velocity, and the hemodynamic characteristics of regional flow in cerebral arteries.

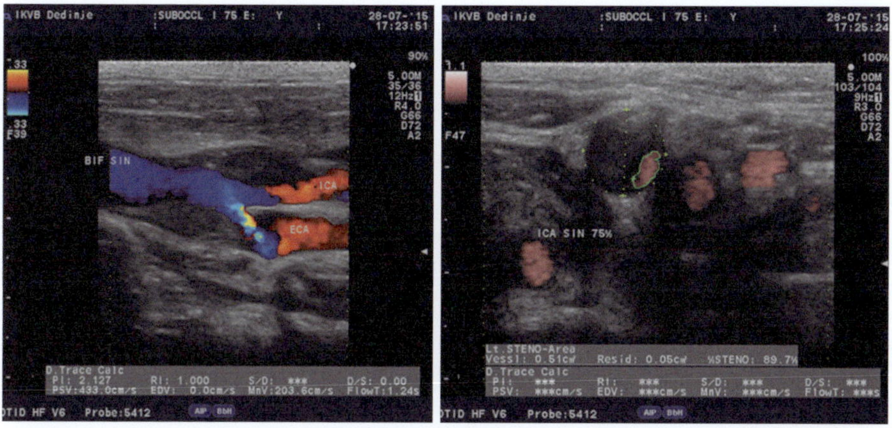

Fig. 4.17 Color and power Doppler flow imaging showing significant internal carotid stenosis

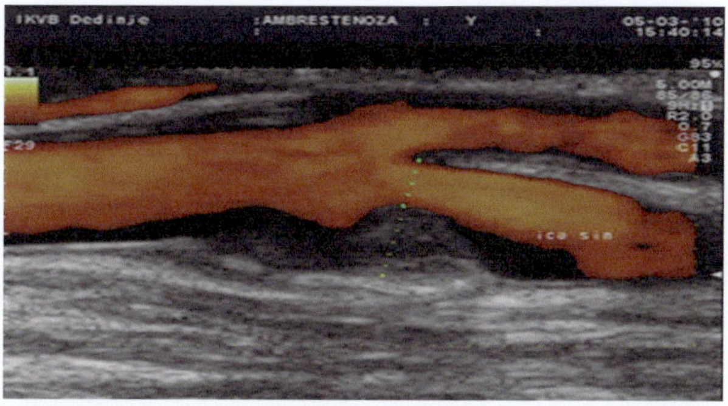

Fig. 4.18 Power Doppler flow analysis showing homogeneous moderate plaque in the internal carotid artery

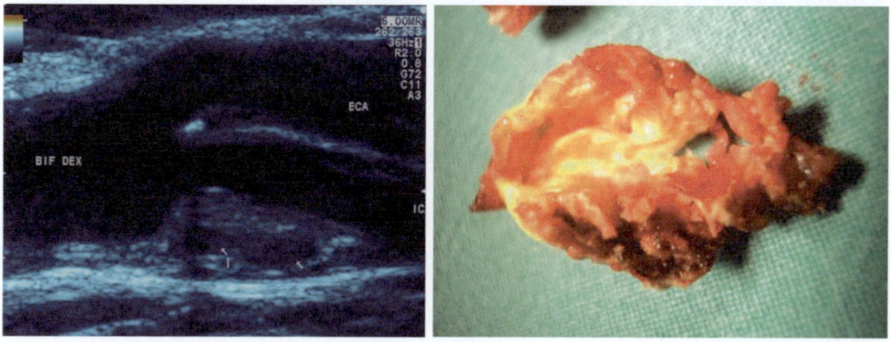

Fig. 4.19 Asymptomatic ulcerated calcified plaque in the form of a "coral reef," with a higher potential for embolization

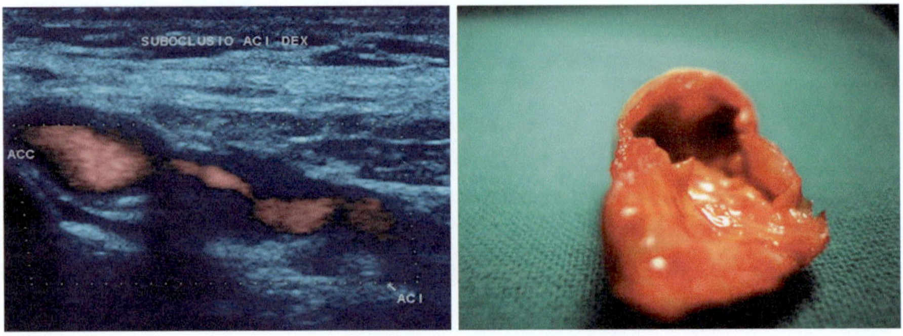

Fig. 4.20 Asymptomatic near-total occlusion with homogeneous fibrous plaque

4.4 Computed Tomography and Magnetic Resonance Angiography

4.4.1 Introduction

Computed Tomography Angiography (CTA) of extracranial and intracranial vessels is a widely available, noninvasive diagnostic modality. Many centers use CTA for all patients with carotid stenosis to obtain a comprehensive assessment of both extra- and intracranial vascular status before making treatment decisions. CTA is a rapid examination that requires intravenous contrast and, with postprocessing software, provides all the necessary information for vascular surgeons within a few minutes. CTA has high sensitivity and specificity, reaching up to 96% and 98%, respectively [10]. Multiplanar reconstructions allow the examination of carotid and vertebral arteries in the axial, sagittal, and coronal planes. Additionally, specialized techniques such as curved planar reconstruction and 3D volume rendering assist vascular surgeons in making informed decisions.

Stenosis measurement on CTA can be performed using two primary methods:

1. **The North American Symptomatic Carotid Endarterectomy Trial (NASCET) method** (Fig. 4.21), which uses the formula (A − B)/A × 100.
2. **The European Carotid Surgery Trial (ECST) method** (Fig. 4.22), which uses the formula (B − A)/B × 100 [11].

4.4.2 Computed Tomography Angiography of Carotid Artery

Computed Tomography Angiography (CTA) provides excellent spatial resolution and high-quality images using iodinated contrast agents. The standard field of view for evaluating carotid artery diseases typically includes the aortic arch, neck, and intracranial segments. CTA is performed with 0.625 mm reconstructions, and contrast is administered through the cubital vein. A small amount of contrast, along with pre-test calculations, helps determine the optimal timing for acquiring high-quality images.

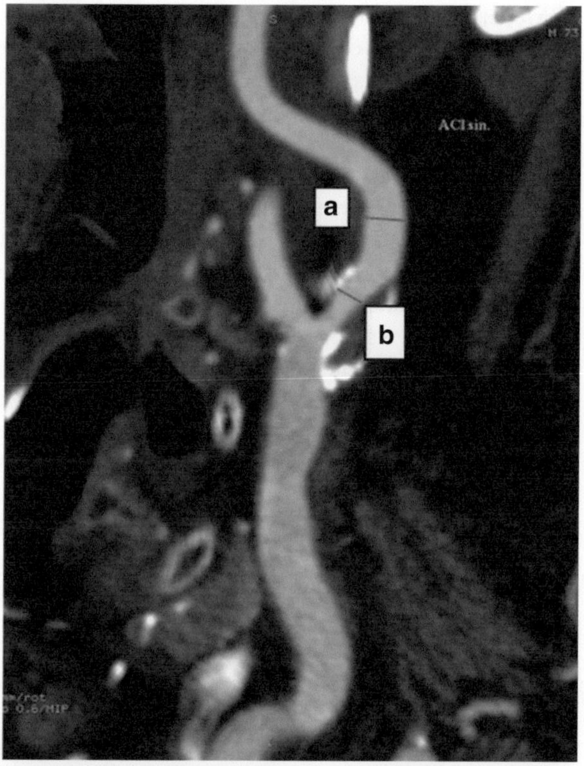

Fig. 4.21 The North American Symptomatic Carotid Endarterectomy Trial (NASCET) stenosis measurement method: (A − B)/A × 100

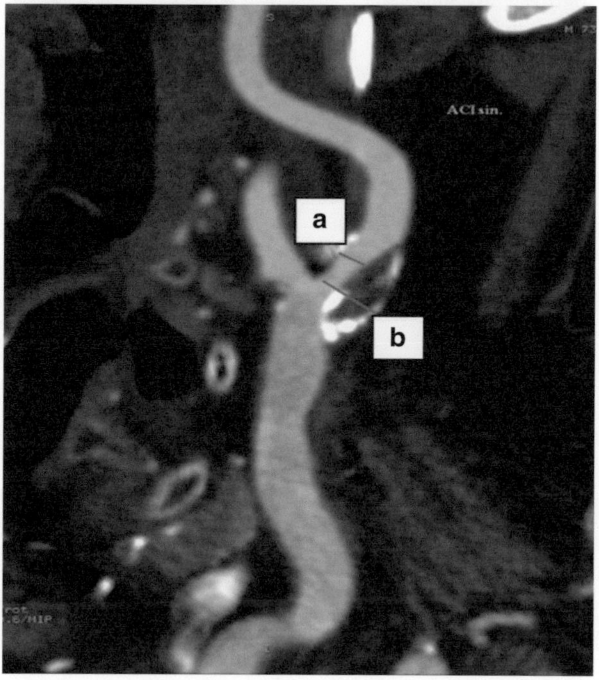

Fig. 4.22 The European Carotid Surgery Trial (ECST) stenosis measurement method: B − A/B × 100

Modern CTA software offers advanced imaging processing and analysis, allowing precise evaluation of carotid arteries. Continuous improvements in software and automated image analysis enable the rapid acquisition of detailed information on plaque characteristics, degree of stenosis, and other relevant conditions in the carotid artery.

However, CTA has drawbacks, including radiation exposure and the potential impact of iodinated contrast on renal function, particularly in patients with pre-existing renal impairment. Although allergic reactions to contrast are rare, proper pre-medication can mitigate risks and allow most patients to be scanned safely.

In clinical practice, vascular surgeons use CTA to assess significant stenosis or occlusion of the aortic arch and supra-aortic vessels, which can influence treatment decisions (Fig. 4.23). CTA also provides critical information on carotid artery lumen analysis, stenosis assessment, and plaque characteristics (Fig. 4.24). It helps evaluate the degree and length of stenosis in the internal carotid artery and identifies any notable intracranial findings, such as stenosis, occlusion, aneurysm, or dissection (Figs. 4.25 and 4.26).

Standard image analysis includes axial, sagittal, coronal, and curved multiplanar reconstructions, as well as 3D vessel rendering. High-risk plaques and thrombi are easily detectable on CTA images (Figs. 4.27 and 4.28) and can influence surgical strategies. In acute stroke diagnosis, advanced perfusion imaging is a significant development, providing rapid assessment for thrombolysis or endovascular thrombectomy (Fig. 4.29). Non-contrast images are used to diagnose or exclude intracerebral hemorrhage (Fig. 4.30).

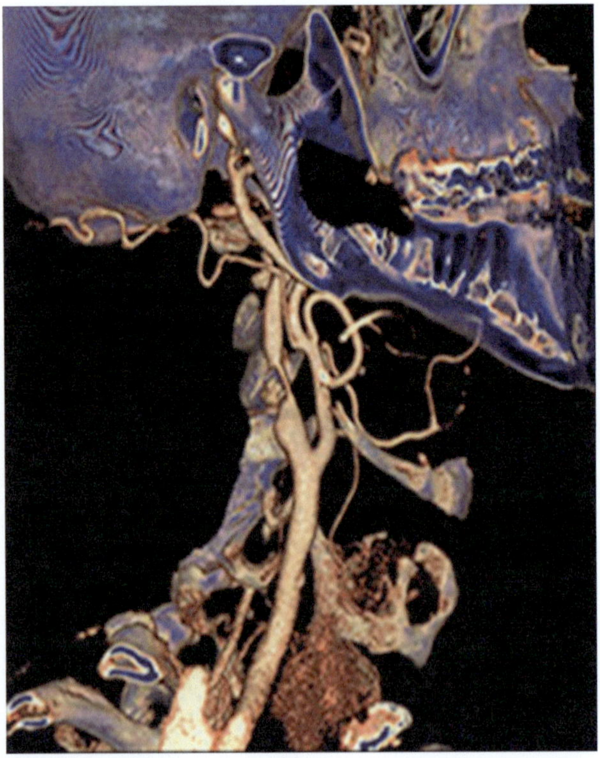

Fig. 4.23 3D volume rendering reconstruction showing internal carotid artery stenosis, indicating suitability for carotid endarterectomy

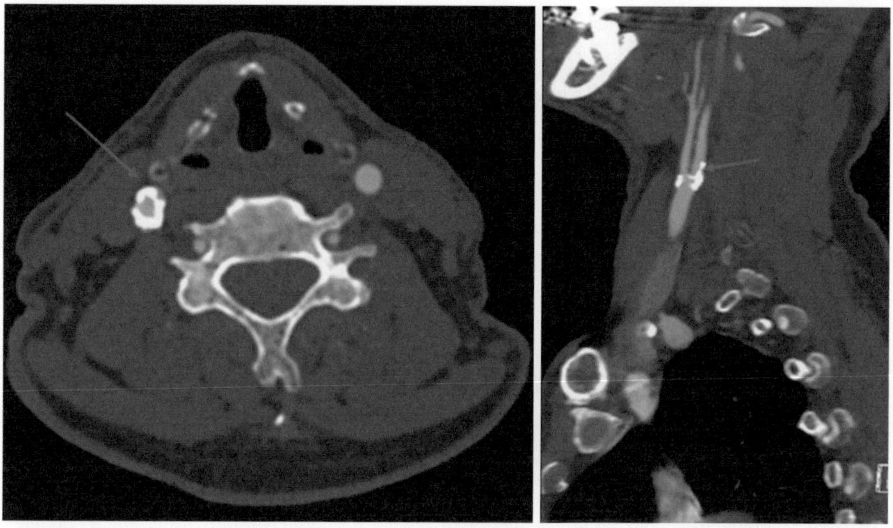

Fig. 4.24 CTA findings reveal ring calcifications and moderate stenosis in the right carotid artery, including the bulb and internal carotid artery, as shown in the axial and sagittal reconstructions (arrows)

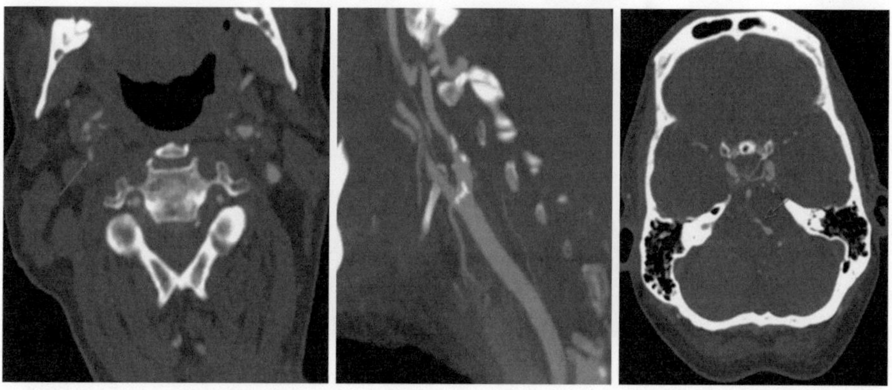

Fig. 4.25 Axial and sagittal reconstructions show significant stenosis of the right internal carotid artery (arrows). An axial image also incidentally reveals an asymptomatic basilar artery aneurysm (arrow)

4.4.3 Magnetic Resonance Angiography

Magnetic Resonance Angiography (MRA) is an advanced, noninvasive diagnostic modality that does not use ionizing radiation and is widely employed for diagnosing vascular diseases with high sensitivity and specificity. Compared to invasive angiography, MRA shows high sensitivity and specificity, reaching up to 93–94% for severe carotid stenosis and occlusion, and 66–93% for moderate carotid stenosis [12]. Generally, two types of angiography modalities are used: non-contrast MRI

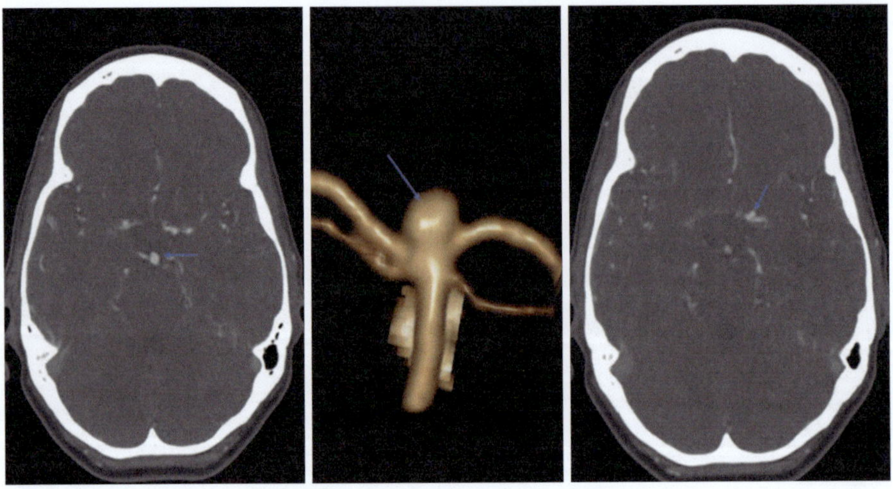

Fig. 4.26 Incidentally, a basilar artery aneurysm and a left middle cerebral artery aneurysm were discovered during the CTA investigation for extracranial carotid artery stenosis

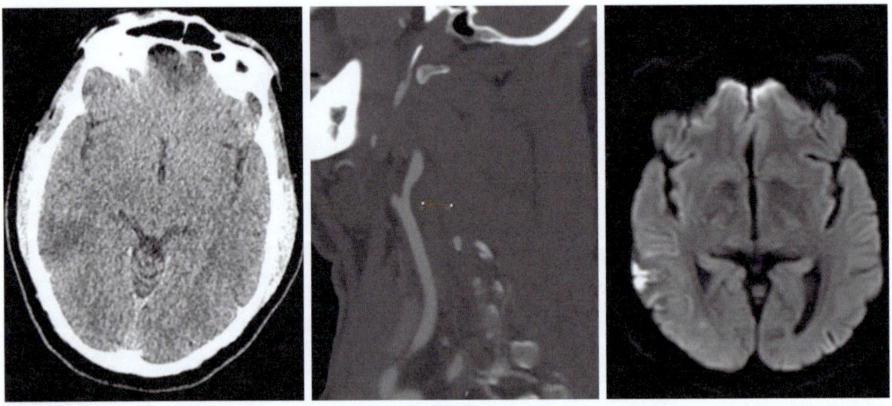

Fig. 4.27 Sagittal projection shows right carotid artery stenosis (arrow) with non-significant stenosis and "unstable" soft plaque. Distal embolization and infarct in the right temporal region are evident on CT and MRI imaging

and contrast-enhanced MRI. Non-contrast MRI techniques include Time of Flight (TOF) (Fig. 4.31), Phase Contrast (PC), and Steady-State Free Precession (SSFP). Contrast-enhanced MRI involves the administration of gadolinium-based contrast (Fig. 4.32).

Non-contrast techniques can be adequate for assessing large vessels like the aorta, but gadolinium contrast is typically required for a definitive and precise diagnosis of smaller vessels such as the carotid and vertebral arteries. Non-contrast methods may either overestimate or underestimate stenosis in branch vessels due to various artifacts during imaging acquisition and processing.

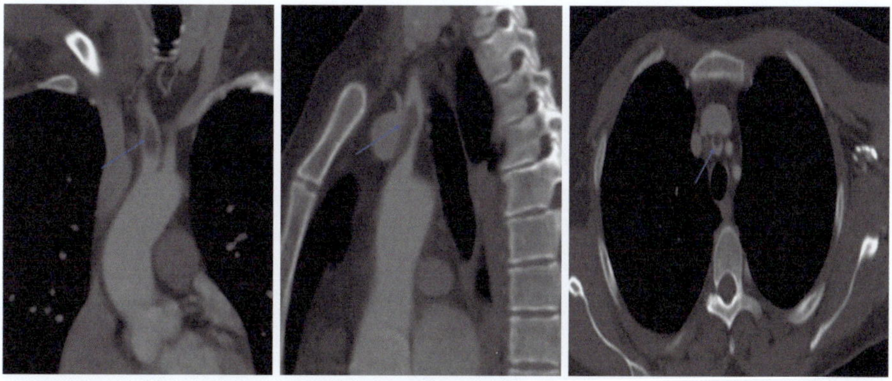

Fig. 4.28 The thrombus in the right brachiocephalic artery, which has a high embolic potential, is easily visible on CTA across different reconstructions (arrows)

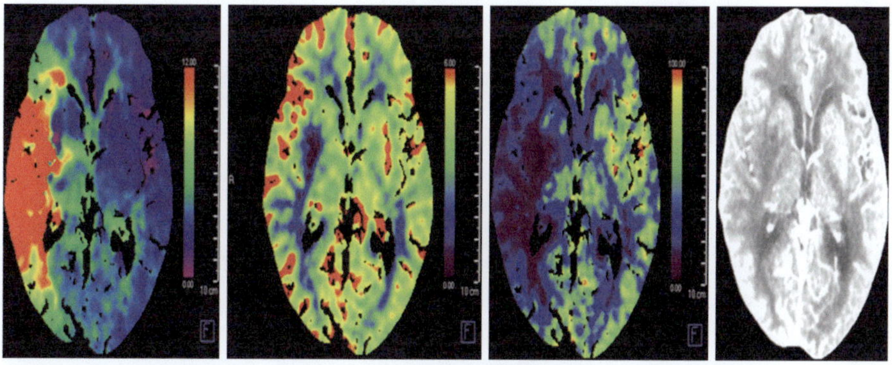

Fig. 4.29 Advanced perfusion sequences in acute stroke allow for the measurement of cerebral volume, blood flow, and mean transit time, with all information obtained within a few minutes

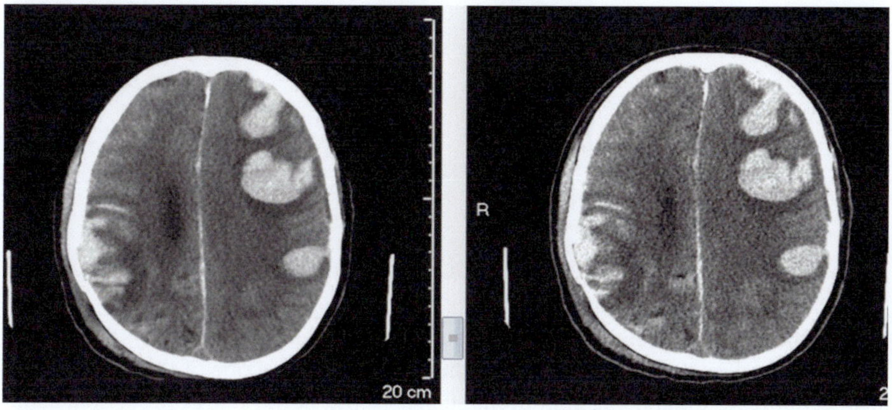

Fig. 4.30 Axial non-contrast cerebral images reveal bleeding in both hemispheres

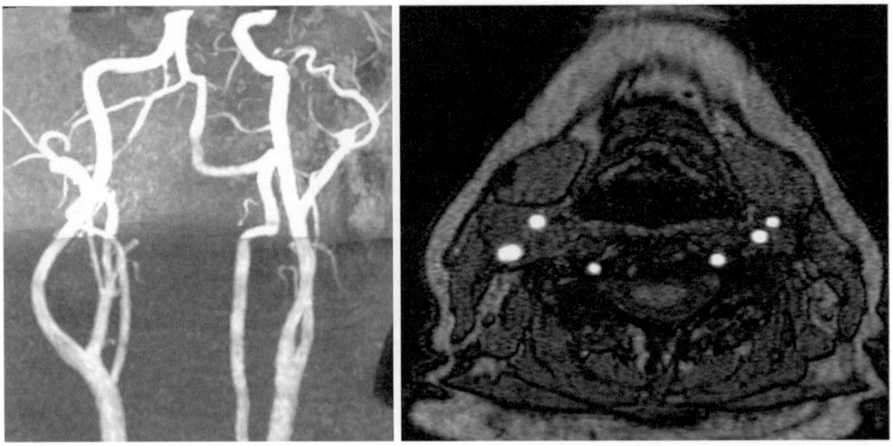

Fig. 4.31 Time of Flight (TOF) non-contrast angiography showing normal carotid and vertebral arteries

Fig. 4.32 Contrast-enhanced MRI of the aortic arch and supra-aortic arteries

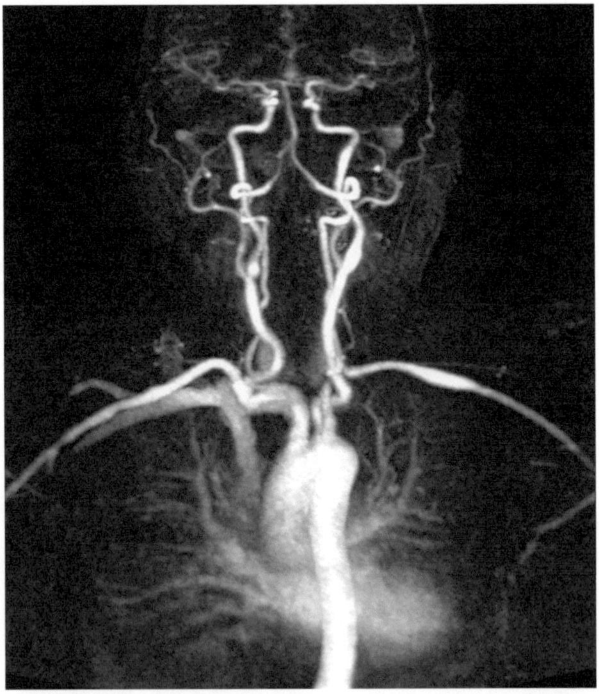

Advanced MRI sequences provide detailed vessel and plaque analysis in multiple planes and reconstructions, though this is beyond the scope of this text. MRI is also valuable for diagnosing conditions such as supra-aortic vessel dissection, aneurysm, carotid tumors, and vasculitis (Fig. 4.33).

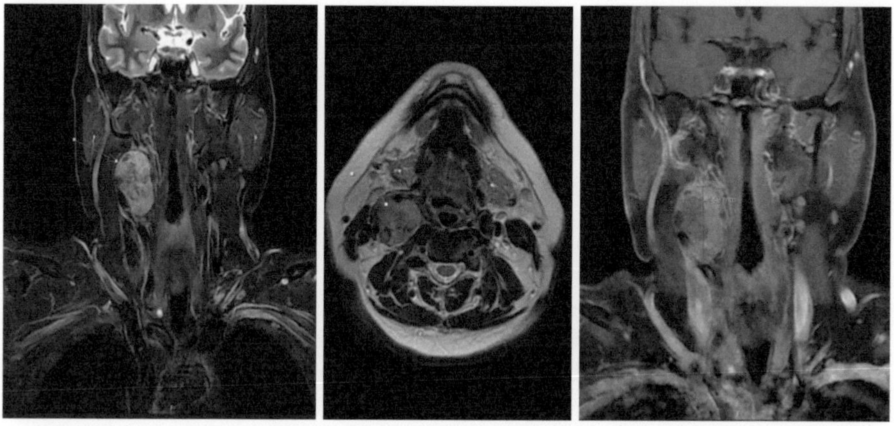

Fig. 4.33 Coronal and axial MRI images of a right carotid body tumor (arrows)

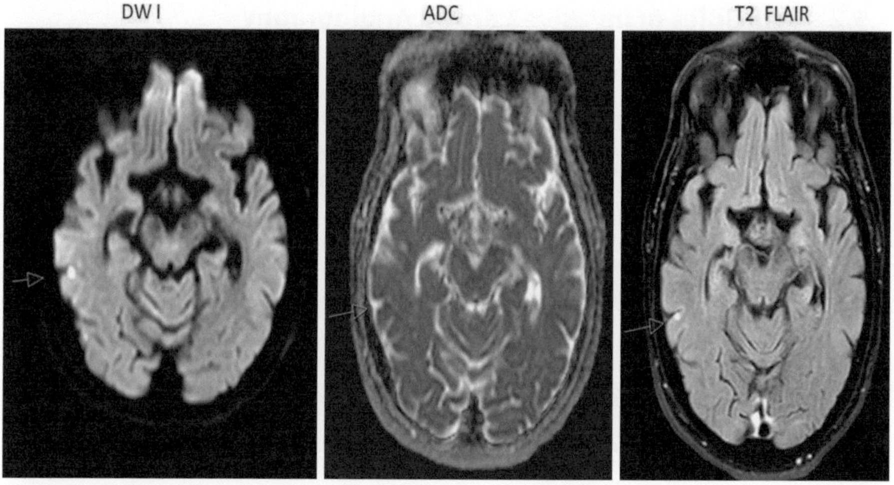

Fig. 4.34 Diffusion-weighted imaging (DWI), Apparent Diffusion Coefficient (ADC), and Fluid Attenuated Inversion Recovery (FLAIR) sequences are used to diagnose stroke. Arrows indicate subacute/chronic stroke in the right temporal region

Similar to CTA, contrast-enhanced MRI uses a test bolus of contrast to optimize the timing of the scan for the best vessel contrast opacification. Caution is needed in patients with severe renal insufficiency due to the risk of nephrogenic systemic fibrosis. MRI is particularly effective for acute stroke diagnosis and other intracranial brain conditions, facilitating prompt treatment (Fig. 4.34).

4.5 Invasive Angiography

4.5.1 Introduction

Invasive cerebral angiography was first introduced in 1927 by Portuguese neurologist Egas Moniz [13]. Initially, invasive angiography was the sole diagnostic method for cerebral vessels. However, advancements in ultrasound, computed tomography, and magnetic resonance imaging have transformed clinical practice. Today, invasive angiography is primarily used as part of the treatment process rather than as a diagnostic tool. Access is typically gained through the femoral or radial/brachial artery. A non-selective angiography catheter, i.e., pigtail catheter (Fig. 4.35) is used for aortography, while various selective diagnostic catheters are employed for selective angiography of the carotid artery (Fig. 4.36).

4.5.2 Principles of Invasive Carotid Angiography

Aortic arch angiography and selective angiography of the supra-aortic branches can be performed through femoral, radial, or brachial artery access. The procedure involves local anesthesia, sterile preparation, and either ultrasound-guided or blind puncture of the artery using a puncture needle. A hydrophilic guidewire, typically 0.035 inches in diameter and 180 cm long, is used for

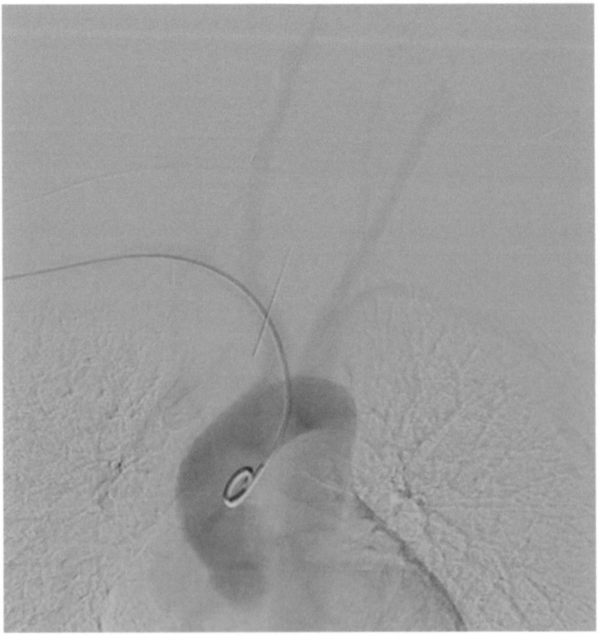

Fig. 4.35 Right radial access with a pigtail catheter for angiography of the aortic arch

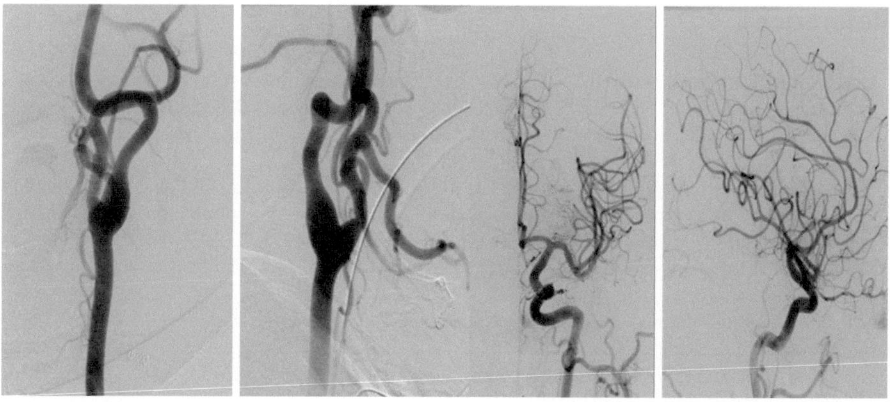

Fig. 4.36 Selective angiography of the carotid artery and intracranial angiography

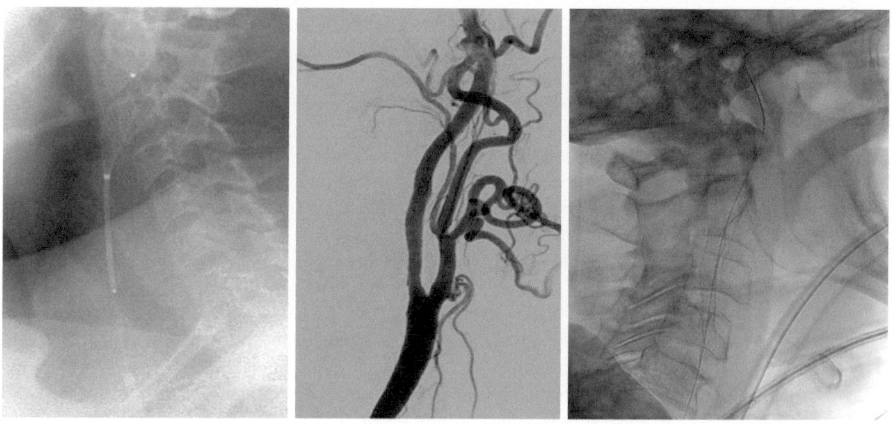

Fig. 4.37 Carotid stent deployment followed by control angiography

angiography, along with a 4 or 5 French (Fr) vascular sheath to secure access. For carotid interventions, longer guidewires (0.014 or 0.018 in.) and a rapid exchange system may also be used. Various 4 or 5 Fr catheters, 90 or 100 cm long, can be advanced through the sheath over the guidewire to perform selective angiography. The carotid artery is optimally visualized in an angled view, typically left or right oblique projection. To prevent distal embolic complications, it is crucial to flush all air from the system before contrast injection and to handle the guidewire and catheter gently. Today, invasive angiography is predominantly used in therapeutic interventions (Fig. 4.37). According to the ACAS study, 1.2% of asymptomatic patients experienced a stroke attributable to angiography, accounting for 50% of all strokes in this group [14]. Other specific local complications during invasive angiography include pseudoaneurysm (>1%), significant hematoma and bleeding (1–3%), dissection, thrombosis, and arteriovenous fistula (0.5%) [15].

References

1. Naylor R, Rantner B, Ancetti S, de Borst GJ, De Carlo M, Halliday A, et al. Editor's choice—European Society for Vascular Surgery (ESVS) 2023 clinical practice guidelines on the management of atherosclerotic carotid and vertebral artery disease. Eur J Vasc Endovasc Surg. 2023;65:7–111.
2. Adams HP Jr, Bendixen BH, Kappelle LJ, Biller J, Love BB, Gordon DL, et al. Classification of subtype of acute ischemic stroke. Definitions for use in a multicenter clinical trial. TOAST. Trial of Org 10172 in Acute Stroke Treatment. Stroke. 1993;24:35–41.
3. Wade DT. Measurement in neurological rehabilitation. New York: Oxford University Press; 1992.
4. Fischer U, Baumgartner A, Arnold M, Nedeltchev K, Gralla J, De Marchis GM, et al. What is a minor stroke? Stroke. 2010;41:661–6.
5. Søren Brostrøm og Niels Saxtrup Nielsen: Subjektivt og Objektivt. Munksgaard Danmark. 1. udgave 3. oplag 2005 s.154–177 3.
6. Paulson og Gjerris et al: Klinisk Neurologi og Neurokirurgi. FADLs forlag. 3. udgave 2001. s. 64.
7. Jahromi AS, Cinà CS, Liu Y, Clase CM. Sensitivity and specificity of color duplex ultrasound measurement in estimating internal carotid artery stenosis: a systematic review and meta-analysis. J Vasc Surg. 2005;41:962–72.
8. AF AR, Srivastava M, Stone PA, Mousa AY, Jain A, Dean LS, et al. Critical appraisal of the Carotid Duplex Consensus criteria in diagnosing carotid artery stenosis. J Vasc Surg. 2011;53:53–9; discussion 59–60.
9. Society for Vascular Ultrasound (SVU). Vascular Technology Professional Performance Guidelines: Extracranial Cerebrovascular Duplex Ultrasound; January 2019.
10. Koelemay MJ, Nederkoorn PJ, Reitsma JB, Majoie CB. Systematic review of computed tomographic angiography for assessment of carotid artery disease. Stroke. 2004;35:2306–12.
11. Donnan GA, Davis SM, Chambers BR, Gates PC. Surgery for prevention of stroke. Lancet. 1998;351:1372–3.
12. Debrey SM, Yu H, Lynch JK, Lövblad KO, Wright VL, Janket SJ, Baird AE. Diagnostic accuracy of magnetic resonance angiography for internal carotid artery disease: a systematic review and meta-analysis. Stroke. 2008;39:2237–48.
13. Artico M, Spoletini M, Fumagalli L, Biagioni F, Ryskalin L, Fornai F, et al. Egas Moniz: 90 Years (1927–2017) from Cerebral Angiography. Front Neuroanat. 2017;19(11):81.
14. Executive Committee for the Asymptomatic Carotid Atherosclerosis Study. Endarterectomy for asymptomatic carotid artery stenosis. JAMA. 1995;273:1421–8.
15. Waugh JR, Sacharias N. Arteriographic complications in the DSA era. Radiology. 1992;182:243–6.

5 Conservative Medical Treatment

Stevo Duvnjak and Djordje Radak

5.1 Introduction

Atherosclerosis is a slow, progressive disease that accelerates with aging, resulting in the thickening, tearing, and eventual complete blockage of arteries supplying various tissues. It starts with the accumulation of lipids and cholesterol, which over time leads to arterial narrowing due to calcium buildup. This process causes ischemia and can lead to thrombus formation, potentially resulting in embolic complications [1]. **Primary prevention** of ischemic stroke involves identifying, eliminating, and managing risk factors in the general population before symptoms occur. **Secondary prevention** focuses on preventing recurrent strokes in patients who have already experienced one, such as those with residual neurological deficits or transient ischemic attacks (TIAs) [2]. Each individual has a specific genetic predisposition that influences the rate of atherosclerosis progression, but this can be modified through preventive measures. Atherosclerosis can be slowed and managed effectively. Since early-stage atherosclerosis often causes no symptoms, preventive measures should be a key focus of patient education. Conservative treatment involves addressing risk factors and medical management. Following successful surgical intervention for carotid artery disease, ongoing conservative treatment should continue with lifestyle modifications and medication.

S. Duvnjak (✉)
Department of Vascular Surgery, Rigshospitalet, Copenhagen, Denmark
e-mail: stevo.duvnjak@regionh.dk

D. Radak
Serbian Academy of Sciences and Arts, Belgrade, Serbia

Clinic for Surgery, Euromedik Hospital, Belgrade, Serbia
e-mail: radak@ikvbd.com

D. Radak, S. Duvnjak (eds.), *Carotid Artery Disease: Surgical Perspectives*, https://doi.org/10.1007/978-3-031-81842-4_5

Lifestyle changes include:

- **Smoking cessation**: Quit smoking to reduce cardiovascular risk.
- **Stress management**: Focus on improving aspects of life within your control.
- **Adequate hydration**: Drink more than 1.5 L of water daily.
- **Healthy diet**: Consume a diet rich in vegetables, unsaturated fats (e.g., fish, seafood, nuts), and omega-3 fatty acids.
- **Limit intake of**: Sugar, saturated animal fats (e.g., fatty meat, cheeses, milk), margarine, fast food, artificial juices, and carbonated drinks.
- **Regular physical activity**: Engage in at least 30 min of exercise or walking daily.
- **Weight management**: Maintain a healthy body weight.
- **Management of chronic conditions**: Regularly treat hypertension, diabetes, and metabolic syndrome.

5.2 Antiplatelet Medications

5.2.1 Mechanism of Acts

Thrombocytes (platelets) in normal circulation are typically inactive and ellipsoidal, playing a crucial role in hemostasis. They release various vasoactive and prothrombotic mediators that promote coagulation in response to endothelial damage, such as that caused by plaque formation, surgery, or vascular interventions [3]. **Antiplatelet drugs** affect platelet activation and aggregation, thereby preventing clot formation.

Acetylsalicylic acid (aspirin) possesses anti-inflammatory, antiplatelet, and analgesic effects, making it one of the most commonly prescribed medications for secondary stroke prevention. Its antithrombotic effect stems from the irreversible inhibition of the cyclooxygenase enzyme, which is essential for the synthesis of prostaglandins and thromboxane. A low dose of 75–150 mg is effective for this purpose. Acetylsalicylic acid irreversibly blocks thromboxane A2 in platelets, thereby preventing platelet activation, aggregation, and adhesion [4].

Thienopyridine drugs, such as clopidogrel, prasugrel, and ticlopidine inhibit adenosine diphosphate (ADP)-mediated platelet activation and clotting. These medications also have indirect antithrombotic effects, including reducing platelet adhesion, lowering plasma fibrinogen levels, and decreasing blood viscosity [5].

Phosphodiesterase inhibitors, such as cilostazol and **dipyridamole**, affect platelet activation and promote vasodilation by modulating platelet receptors, increasing cyclic adenosine monophosphate (cAMP) levels, and inhibiting phosphodiesterase [6].

Glycoprotein platelet inhibitors, such as Abciximab, tirofiban, and **eptifibatide,** block glycoprotein IIb/IIIa platelet receptors, thereby decreasing platelet aggregation. These drugs are used parenterally for acute coronary, peripheral, and central endovascular thrombosis treatments [7].

Performing a platelet reactivity test is highly useful for selecting the most effective antiplatelet drug for a patient, based on their individual genetic expression and receptor response [8].

5.2.2 Doses and Duration of Treatment

Initiating acetylsalicylic acid monotherapy as quickly as possible in a patient who has experienced an ischemic episode is crucial. This approach can reduce the risk of recurrent stroke by up to 60% and decrease the likelihood of disabling or fatal recurrent stroke by up to 70% compared to a placebo [9].

The European Society for Vascular Surgery, in guidelines published in 2023, recommends the following [10, 11].

- **Patients with asymptomatic >50% carotid artery stenosis:** Low-dose acetylsalicylic acid (75–325 mg) is recommended to reduce the risk of secondary cardiovascular events.
- **Patients with asymptomatic >50% stenosis and acetylsalicylic acid intolerance:** Clopidogrel 75 mg or dipyridamole 200 mg twice daily is recommended.
- **Patients with transient ischemic attack or minor ischemic stroke and any degree of carotid stenosis, not undergoing carotid endarterectomy or stenting:** Dual antiplatelet therapy with aspirin (75–325 mg) and clopidogrel (75 mg) is recommended for 21 days, followed by clopidogrel 75 mg or long-term aspirin (75–100 mg) plus dipyridamole (200 mg twice daily) to reduce stroke risk.
- **Recently symptomatic patients undergoing carotid endarterectomy:** Dual antiplatelet therapy with aspirin (75–325 mg) and clopidogrel (75 mg) should be considered peri-operatively to reduce recurrent stroke risk.
- **Patients with ischemic cerebral events, both undergoing and not undergoing carotid intervention:** Long-term dual antiplatelet therapy with aspirin and clopidogrel is not recommended, as it does not confer additional benefit over single antiplatelet therapy and increases bleeding risk.
- **Patients with asymptomatic carotid stenosis undergoing carotid stenting:** Combination antiplatelet therapy with aspirin (75–325 mg daily) and clopidogrel (75 mg daily) is recommended. Clopidogrel (75 mg daily) should be started at least 3 days before stenting or as a single 300 mg loading dose in urgent cases. Continue aspirin and clopidogrel for at least 4 weeks post-stenting, then switch to indefinite antiplatelet monotherapy.

5.3 Non-vitamin K Oral Anticoagulants—NOACs

5.3.1 Mechanism of Acts

Non-vitamin K oral anticoagulants (NOACs) work through direct inhibition of specific coagulation factors:

- **Rivaroxaban, Apixaban, and Edoxaban**: These NOACs directly inhibit Factor Xa, a key component in the coagulation cascade that plays a central role in thrombin generation.

- **Dabigatran**: This NOAC directly inhibits thrombin (Factor IIa), which is crucial in the final steps of coagulation.

A key advantage of NOACs over traditional vitamin K antagonists (e.g., warfarin) is that they do not require routine monitoring of coagulation parameters, making them more convenient for patients [12]. Patients with renal and liver impairment require reduced doses, or in severe cases, medications are contraindicated.

5.3.2 Doses and Duration of Treatment

For stroke prevention in patients with non-valvular atrial fibrillation, the recommended doses of NOACs are as follows:

- **Rivaroxaban**: 20 mg daily (15 mg daily in patients with renal impairment).
- **Apixaban**: 5 mg twice daily (2.5 mg twice daily in patients with renal impairment).
- **Edoxaban**: 60 mg daily (30 mg daily in patients with renal impairment).
- **Dabigatran**: 150 mg twice daily (110 mg twice daily in patients with renal impairment).

NOACs are generally considered non-inferior to vitamin K antagonists (e.g., warfarin) in preventing stroke in patients with atrial fibrillation. They also tend to have a lower risk of major bleeding complications compared to vitamin K antagonists [13]. For secondary stroke prevention in patients with carotid stenosis who do not have atrial fibrillation, recommendations are less standardized. However, some studies have investigated the use of non-vitamin K oral anticoagulants (NOACs) such as rivaroxaban at 2.5 mg twice daily, which has shown potential for stroke reduction but is associated with a higher risk of bleeding complications.

In patients with a mobile thrombus in the aortic arch, the following anticoagulation strategies may be considered, especially if surgery is not feasible:

- **NOACs**: For patients not undergoing surgery, NOACs like rivaroxaban, apixaban, or dabigatran may be used, depending on individual risk factors and the potential for bleeding.
- **Warfarin or Heparin**: These may be used as alternatives, particularly if NOACs are contraindicated or not tolerated.

For patients who need surgical intervention, NOACs are typically paused for 2–3 days before the surgery. In such cases, bridging with heparin is usually not performed unless specifically indicated based on individual bleeding and thromboembolic risks. This approach helps manage the risk of thromboembolism while minimizing the potential for perioperative bleeding (Figs. 5.1 and 5.2).

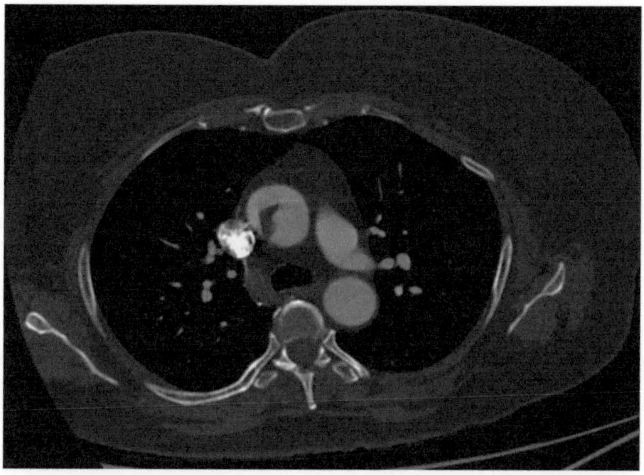

Fig. 5.1 The spontaneous thrombus in the ascending aorta has a high embolic potential. Fortunately, the patient experienced the embolic complications manifested in the right upper extremities, leading to the need for a brachial thrombectomy.

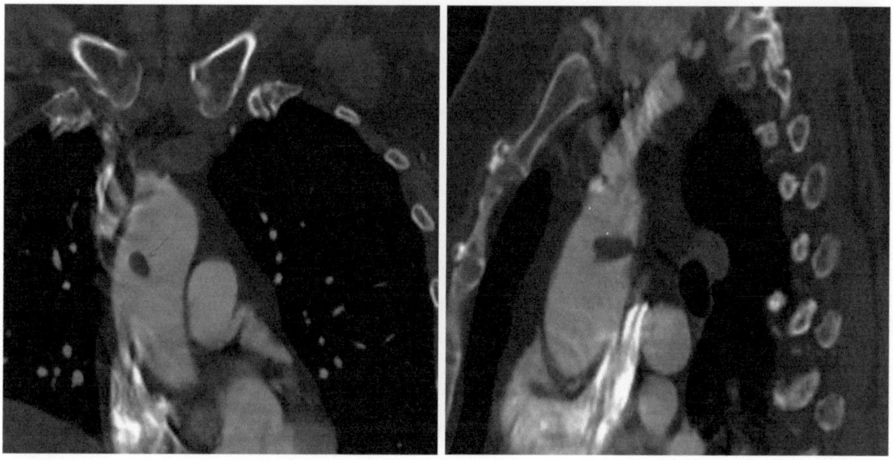

Fig. 5.2 Coronal and sagittal computed tomography reconstruction revealed a spontaneous thrombus in the ascending aorta, which was conservatively treated with anticoagulant medications

5.4 Lipid-Lowering Therapy—Statin

5.4.1 Mechanism of Acts

The discovery of statins (3-hydroxy-3-methylglutaryl coenzyme A–HMG-CoA reductase inhibitors) has significantly improved the treatment of cardiovascular morbidity and dyslipidemia. A large meta-analysis demonstrated that for each mmol/L decrease in low-density lipoprotein (LDL) cholesterol, statin drugs reduce the risk of any major cardiovascular event by 21% and decrease the risk of both fatal and non-fatal stroke by up to 12% [14]. Statins reduce cholesterol biosynthesis primarily in the liver by inhibiting HMG-CoA reductase. Additionally, statins have been shown to decrease perioperative mortality and morbidity in vascular surgery, as confirmed by various studies [15]. Statins reduce intima-media thickness and microembolization in the carotid arteries of asymptomatic patients [16].

Atorvastatin, lovastatin, pravastatin, rosuvastatin, fluvastatin, and simvastatin are first-choice drugs for treating dyslipidemia. Dyslipidemia is also managed through diet and physical activity. The target value for total cholesterol is <4 mmol/L (175 mg/dL), and for LDL cholesterol, it is below 2.6 mmol/L (100 mg/dL), with a target of <1.8 mmol/L for high-risk patients. Meta-analysis of secondary stroke prevention has confirmed a significant reduction in stroke risk among patients taking statins. However, there was no statistically significant difference in primary stroke prevention between patients who took statins and those who did not [17].

Other drugs used to treat dyslipidemia include fibrate derivatives, nicotinic acid, ion exchange resins, medications that lower triglyceride levels, and cholesterol absorption inhibitors.

Statins also have cholesterol-independent pleiotropic effects that help reduce the inflammatory components of metabolic processes within the arterial wall. Their mechanisms of action include:

- Increased expression of nitric oxide synthase, leading to enhanced production of nitric oxide (NO) and repair of endothelial dysfunction.
- Reduction in the adhesion of leukocytes and macrophages to the endothelium, along with immunomodulation.
- Decrease in endothelial cell apoptosis.
- Increase in apoptosis of smooth muscle cells.
- Reduction in the proliferation of smooth muscle cells within the plaque.
- Decrease in the activity of local macrophages and the production of metalloproteinases [18].

5.4.2 Doses and Duration of Treatment

Atorvastatin 80 mg daily is typically the first-line treatment for hypercholesterolemia. If hypercholesterolemia proves resistant to atorvastatin, ezetimibe (a cholesterol absorption inhibitor) 10 mg can be added. New medications, such as PCSK9 inhibitors, are also showing promising results in the treatment of hypercholesterolemia.

5.5 Antihypertensive Medications

5.5.1 Mechanism of Acts

There are various antihypertensive medications available. The most commonly recommended first-line treatments are thiazide diuretics, angiotensin-converting enzyme (ACE) inhibitors, and calcium channel blockers. Beta-blockers are generally not recommended as first-line therapy.

The primary mechanism of action of thiazide diuretics is their ability to inhibit the reabsorption of sodium and chloride from the distal renal tubule, which contributes to their antihypertensive effect [19].

Angiotensin-converting enzyme (ACE) inhibitors block the enzyme responsible for converting angiotensin I to angiotensin II. This action enhances natriuresis, lowers blood pressure, and prevents the remodeling of smooth muscle and cardiac myocytes. By reducing arterial and venous pressure, ACE inhibitors decrease both preload and afterload [20].

Calcium channel blockers inhibit calcium uptake into cells, leading to the relaxation of arterial smooth muscle and subsequent dilation of arteries, which lowers blood pressure [21].

5.5.2 Doses and Duration of Treatment

The guidelines recommend a target blood pressure of <130/80 mmHg for non-diabetic patients under 65 years of age, and <140/80 mmHg for non-diabetic patients aged 65 and older. For diabetic patients, the target blood pressure is 120–129/70–79 mmHg for those under 65 years of age, and 130–139/70–79 mmHg for those aged 65 and older [10, 17].

5.6 Heparin and Warfarin Medication

5.6.1 Mechanism of Acts

Heparin is one of the oldest and most widely used anticoagulants in medicine and belongs to the glycosaminoglycan family [22]. There are different types of heparin:

- **Unfractionated heparin** is a sulfated glycosaminoglycan with an average molecular weight of 15,000–19,000 Daltons (Da). Its bioactivity and actions are more unpredictable compared to low molecular weight heparin.
- **Low molecular weight heparin (LMWH)**, such as enoxaparin, dalteparin, and tinzaparin, has a molecular weight of 3000–6500 Da. It offers better bioavailability and more predictable action. LMWH can be administered in an outpatient setting and does not require routine monitoring.
- **Ultra-low molecular weight heparin (ULMWH)** has a molecular weight of less than 3000 Da. Due to its higher cost, it is not widely used in practice.

The anticoagulant effect of heparin is based on increased activity of antithrombin and the mobilization of tissue factor pathway inhibitors. Antithrombin III inhibits thrombin, factor Xa, and other components of the coagulation cascade, thereby preventing clot formation. Tissue factor pathway inhibitors prevent the conversion of factor X to Xa and factor IX to IXa [23].

Activated partial thromboplastin time (aPTT) is used to monitor unfractionated heparin therapy, while low molecular weight heparin (LMWH) does not require routine monitoring.

Warfarin is the most commonly used oral anticoagulant. Its anticoagulant effect is based on the inhibition of vitamin K epoxide reductase, an enzyme necessary for the reactivation of vitamin K1. Without this reactivation, the plasma concentrations of coagulation factors II, VII, IX, and X are reduced, leading to decreased coagulation capability [24].

5.6.2 Doses and Duration of Treatment

Heparin doses for carotid surgery typically range from 70 to 100 units/kg administered before clamping the artery. Warfarin therapy usually begins with a dose of 5 mg (or 2.5 mg in high-risk patients), with the therapeutic effect expected to be achieved within 4–5 days. Prothrombin time is monitored using the International Normalized Ratio (INR), which should be assessed before starting warfarin and again after 4 days to ensure proper management. The target INR values are between 2.0 and 3.0. Warfarin should be discontinued 3–5 days prior to surgery. If needed, INR values can be normalized during surgery using low molecular weight heparin as bridging therapy.

Postoperatively, the patient should resume standard oral anticoagulant therapy on the second day and discontinue low molecular weight heparin on the same day.

References

1. Weber C, Noels H. Atherosclerosis: current pathogenesis and therapeutic options. Nat Med. 2011;17:1410–22.
2. Caprio FZ, Sorond FA. Cerebrovascular disease: primary and secondary stroke prevention. Med Clin North Am. 2019;103:295–308.
3. Davì G, Patrono C. Platelet activation and atherothrombosis. N Engl J Med. 2007;357:2482–94.
4. Burch JW, Stanford N, Majerus PW. Inhibition of platelet prostaglandin synthetase by oral aspirin. J Clin Invest. 1978;61:314–9.
5. Lubbe DF, Berger PB. The thienopyridines. J Interv Cardiol. 2002;15:85–93.
6. Shah J, Liu S, Yu W. Contemporary antiplatelet therapy for secondary stroke prevention: a narrative review of current literature and guidelines. Stroke Vasc Neurol. 2022;7:406–14.
7. Lefkovits J, Plow EF, Topol EJ. Platelet glycoprotein IIb/IIIa receptors in cardiovascular medicine. N Engl J Med. 1995;332:1553–9.
8. Erdman MK, Leary MC. Antiplatelet agents. Primer on cerebrovascular diseases. 2nd ed. Cambridge, MA: Academic Press; 2017.
9. Rothwell PM, Algra A, Chen Z, Diener HC, Norrving B, Mehta Z. Effects of aspirin on risk and severity of early recurrent stroke after transient ischaemic attack and ischaemic stroke: time-course analysis of randomised trials. Lancet. 2016;23(388):365–75.
10. Naylor R, Rantner B, Ancetti S, de Borst GJ, De Carlo M, Halliday A, et al. Editor's choice—European Society for Vascular Surgery (ESVS) 2023 Clinical Practice Guidelines on the management of atherosclerotic carotid and vertebral artery disease. Eur J Vasc Endovasc Surg. 2023;65:7–111.

11. Twine CP, Kakkos SK, Aboyans V, Baumgartner I, Behrendt CA, Bellmunt-Montoya S, et al. Editor's choice—European Society for Vascular Surgery (ESVS) 2023 Clinical Practice Guidelines on antithrombotic therapy for vascular diseases. Eur J Vasc Endovasc Surg. 2023;65:627–89.
12. Del Brutto VJ, Chaturvedi S, Diener HC, Romano JG, Sacco RL. Antithrombotic therapy to prevent recurrent strokes in ischemic cerebrovascular disease: JACC Scientific Expert Panel. J Am Coll Cardiol. 2019;74:786–803.
13. Chen A, Stecker E, Warden A, B. Direct oral anticoagulant use: a practical guide to common clinical challenges. J Am Heart Assoc. 2020;9:e017559.
14. Paraskevas KI, Hamilton G, Mikhailidis DP. Statins: an essential component in the management of carotid artery disease. J Vasc Surg. 2007;46:373–86.
15. Paraskevas KI, Mikhailidis DP, Veith FJ. Optimal statin type and dosage for vascular patients. J Vasc Surg. 2011;53:837–44.
16. Baigent C, Keech A, Kearney PM, Blackwell L, Buck G, Pollicino CK, Cholesterol Treatment Trialists' (CTT) Collaborators, et al. Efficacy and safety of cholesterol-lowering treatment: prospective meta-analysis of data from 90,056 participants in 14 randomised trials of statins. Lancet. 2005;366:1267–78.
17. Williams B, Mancia G, Spiering W, Agabiti Rosei E, Azizi M, Burnier M, et al. ESC Scientific Document Group. 2018 ESC/ESH Guidelines for the management of arterial hypertension. Eur Heart J. 2018;39:3021–104.
18. Maron DJ, Fazio S, Linton MF. Current perspectives on statins. Circulation. 2000;101:207–13.
19. Anisman SD, Erickson SB, Fodor KM. Thiazide diuretics. BMJ. 2024;384:e075174.
20. Timmermans PB, Wong PC, Chiu AT, Herblin WF, Benfield P, Carini DJ, Lee RJ, Wexler RR, Saye JA, Smith RD. Angiotensin II receptors and angiotensin II receptor antagonists. Pharmacol Rev. 1993;45:205–51.
21. Elliott WJ, Ram CV. Calcium channel blockers. J Clin Hypertens (Greenwich). 2011;13:687–9.
22. Oduah EI, Linhardt RJ, Sharfstein ST. Heparin: past, present, and future. Pharmaceuticals (Basel). 2016;4(9):38.
23. Beurskens DMH, Huckriede JP, Schrijver R, Hemker HC, Reutelingsperger CP, Nicolaes GAF. The anticoagulant and nonanticoagulant properties of heparin. Thromb Haemost. 2020;120:1371–83.
24. Hirsh J, Fuster V, Ansell J, Halperin JL, American Heart Association/American College of Cardiology Foundation. American Heart Association/American College of Cardiology Foundation guide to warfarin therapy. J Am Coll Cardiol. 2003;41:1633–52.

Open Surgical Treatment of Carotid Artery Stenosis

6

Djordje Radak and Stevo Duvnjak

6.1 Introduction

The purpose of carotid reconstruction (including endarterectomy, bypass, or stenting) is to prevent ischemic stroke, eliminate neurological symptoms and complaints, and avert vascular dementia, cognitive disorders, and senility. Effective artery reconstruction involves:

- **Judiciously setting indications for the procedure**
- **Ensuring precision in the technical execution of the operation**

Early diagnosis and treatment of brain ischemia are crucial because carotid disease is often underestimated by the public. It is the only cause of stroke that can be addressed with an intervention that is neither excessively difficult nor highly risky. Additionally, brain ischemia often lacks symptoms that cause discomfort, leading patients to ignore or downplay their symptoms. For a long time, there was a belief that these interventions were too risky, but large clinical studies conducted toward the end of the last century have definitively demonstrated the benefits of brain revascularization. The best outcomes are observed in centers that perform a high volume of procedures annually, where surgeons, anesthesiologists, and all staff are experienced and well-trained.

D. Radak
Serbian Academy of Sciences and Arts, Belgrade, Serbia

Clinic for Surgery, Euromedik Hospital, Belgrade, Serbia
e-mail: radak@ikvbd.com

S. Duvnjak (✉)
Department of Vascular Surgery, Rigshospitalet, Copenhagen, Denmark
e-mail: stevo.duvnjak@regionh.dk

D. Radak, S. Duvnjak (eds.), *Carotid Artery Disease: Surgical Perspectives*,
https://doi.org/10.1007/978-3-031-81842-4_6

When determining the necessity of carotid artery reconstruction, the following factors are considered:

- Severity and frequency of episodes or symptoms of brain ischemia
- Degree of carotid stenosis and morphological characteristics of the plaque
- Acuteness and severity of any definitive brain damage

A preoperative conversation with the patient is neither underestimated nor overemphasized. It helps the patient relax and fosters an atmosphere of trust, thereby enhancing both the patient's and the surgeon's motivation.

The patient must understand:

- The beneficial effects of brain revascularization, such as prevention of stroke, relief of symptoms, and prevention of dementia
- The risks associated with the natural progression of the disease
- The potential complications of the surgical procedure
- The expected quality of life with and without surgery
- How to manage life post-surgery, including hygiene, dietary changes, and medication therapy
- Potential complications associated with the surgery

Carotid artery reconstruction can be performed using the following methods:

- Carotid endarterectomy
- Interposition (bypass) with a graft
- Endovascular procedures (dilatation, stenting, or graft-stenting)

6.2 Open Surgical Treatment of Symptomatic Carotid Stenosis with Standard Endarterectomy Technique

Traditional carotid endarterectomy is performed through a longitudinal incision in the carotid artery. It involves removing the diseased intima and thickened atherosclerotic media. The lamina elastic externa remains exposed, smooth, and clean, which helps preserve the integrity of the artery. The operation can be performed under general anesthesia or local/regional anesthesia. Carotid endarterectomy involves removing atherosclerotic material from the internal, external, and common carotid arteries. The procedure requires precise technique and aims for the shortest possible clamping time. An intraluminal shunt may be used if necessary to ensure adequate brain perfusion during the central part of the operation. Bypass reconstruction of the diseased segment of the artery with a graft is rarely needed. Large international randomized controlled trials have shown that carotid artery reconstruction is highly beneficial and necessary for patients with symptomatic carotid artery stenosis greater than 70% and symptoms of cerebral ischemia. It provides moderate benefit in cases of stenosis between 50% and 70%. The cumulative risk of stroke and ischemic symptoms is reduced by 33% per year in operated patients compared to those who received the best medical therapy, based on 8 years of follow-up.

- **North American Symptomatic Carotid Endarterectomy Trial (NASCET)** [1].
- **European Carotid Surgery Trial (ESCT)** [2].
- **Veterans Administration (VA) Symptomatic Trial** [3].

European Society of Vascular Surgeons published up-to-date guidelines for treating carotid stenosis [4].

- Operative treatment of carotid stenosis is indicated in symptomatic patients with stenosis greater than 70% and probably in patients with stenosis greater than 50% (NASCET).
- Carotid endarterectomy should be performed within 2 weeks of the last symptoms.
- Endarterectomy can be successful even in high-risk patients with good results, with a low rate of postoperative stroke and cardiac complications.
- An acceptable rate of neurological and cardiac complications accompanies endarterectomy in patients older than 80 years.
- In asymptomatic patients with an extremely high risk (several associated severe diseases), the best choice would be medical treatment.

A vascular council, which includes a vascular surgeon, angiologist, neurologist, cardiologist, and anesthesiologist, determines the indications for surgical treatment by considering:

- Localization, character, and degree of the arterial lesion.
- Stage of ischemic brain damage.
- Presence of associated diseases, particularly those posing cardiac risks.

Preoperative preparation of the operative field in the ward should be done thoroughly. The relevant areas should be shaved the day before to minimize the risk of skin lesions. After antiseptic preparation with disinfectant solutions, the operative field should be dried. Sterile compresses and sheets should be used to protect the field from non-sterile environments. Applying a sterile self-adhesive film (sterile drape) helps prevent infection from the patient's skin flora. The sterile prepared area must be sufficiently large to accommodate potential complications and additional incisions (Fig. 6.1).

The position of the patient on the operating table is important because:
- Facilitates or complicates the operation.
- Prevents long-term pressure lesions on nerves and skin due to unnatural positioning.

The primary rule for positioning is that the surgical incision should be made in the highest region of the patient's body. The surgical technique for arterial dissection must be straightforward and precise. This involves entering the appropriate layer by opening the periarterial connective tissue sheath, which helps preserve all

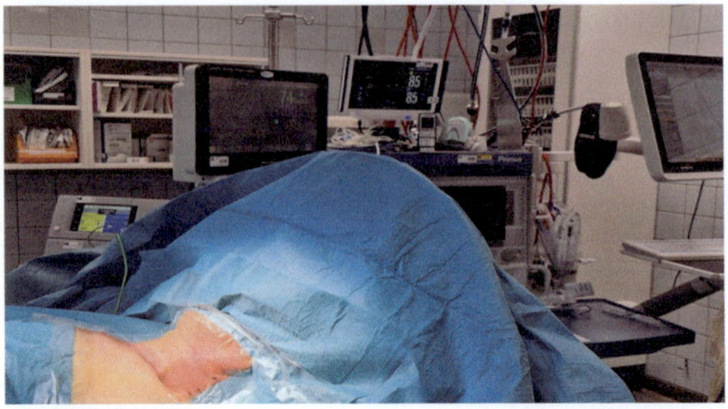

Fig. 6.1 Proper patient positioning and sterile preparation ensure safe and complete exposure of the carotid arteries

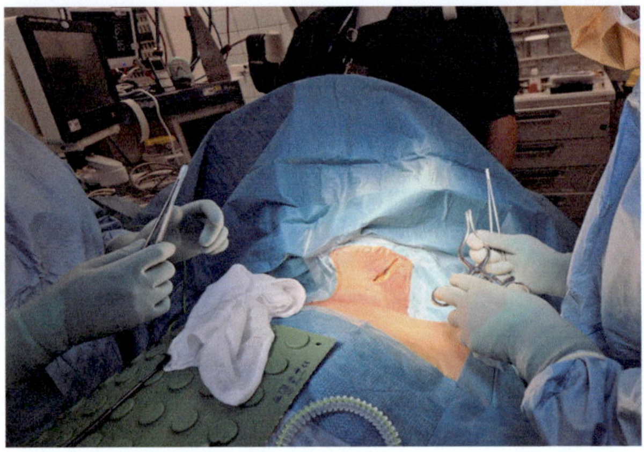

Fig. 6.2 Intraoperative view after making a skin incision along the anterior border of the sternocleidomastoid muscle

surrounding structures. Most surgeons make longitudinal incisions along the anterior border of the sternocleidomastoid muscle and extend the dissection through the platysma to the jugular vein and carotid artery. The entire circumference of the artery is then sharply dissected with scissors, taking care to preserve the side branches and surrounding structures. Arterial trunks are restrained with elastic bands, and lateral branches are dissected carefully. Exposing and restraining the side branches with vessel loops allow for control and temporary interruption of circulation by gentle tightening, rather than clamping.

Surgical exposure of the carotid arteries and supra-aortic branches requires precise and sharp techniques (Figs. 6.2 and 6.3). During manipulation, there is a risk of injuring the surounding nerve and veins.

Rough movements can trigger the detachment of a peripheral thrombus which usually exists in complicated lesions, any disturbance of the plaque can lead to its dislodgment and potential embolization to one of the brain's terminal branches. Therefore, during the dissection of the carotid artery, the plaque should not be touched or moved. Instead, the surrounding tissue should be carefully separated from it without unnecessary manipulation. The principle is that "the patient should be separated from the artery," rather than moving the artery itself. A well-executed vascular reconstruction should result in minimal blood loss and eliminate the need for additional blood.

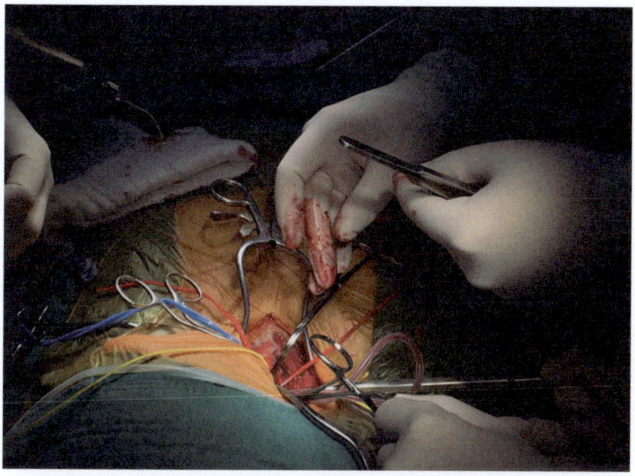

Fig. 6.3 Furthermore, exposeure of the common, external and internal carotid artery and prepare for the endarterectomy

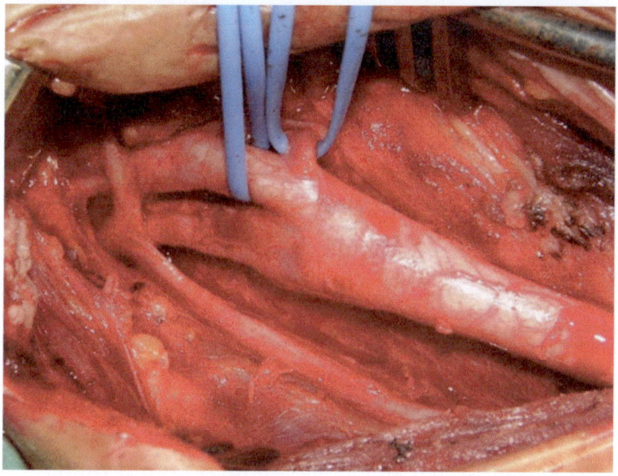

Fig. 6.4 The carotid bifurcation is exposed with vessel loops placed around the superior thyroid and external carotid arteries. Distally, the hypoglossal nerve can be preserved, while the ansa cervicalis crosses the internal carotid artery and the vagus nerve is situated below

The carotid artery is surrounded by cervical and autonomic nerves, including the hypoglossal and vagus nerves, as well as prominent veins. It is essential to preserve these surrounding structures, making precise and delicate surgical exposure crucial (Fig. 6.4).

Clamping of the supra-aortic branches invariably results in some degree of temporary brain ischemia. Therefore, the clamping duration should be kept as brief as possible. If this is not feasible, protection with an intraluminal shunt is necessary. A carefully selected "healthy" arterial segment should be clamped with an atraumatic clamp, applied just enough to occlude the circulation.

6.2.1 Intraoperative Protection Against Brain Ischemia

Intraoperative monitoring of brain perfusion is crucial and includes methods such as transcranial Doppler, stump pressure measurement, near-infrared cerebral oximetry

(NIRS) (Fig. 6.5), and evoked potentials. These techniques help detect intraoperative ischemia during dissection, temporary closure, and clamping.

To prevent intraoperative brain ischemia, an intraluminal shunt can be placed. Near-infrared cerebral spectrophotometry (NIRS) is particularly useful for monitoring brain nutrition. It provides a simple, cost-effective, and reliable means of detecting intraoperative brain ischemia. This optical method measures tissue oxygen saturation in the cerebral cortex (e.g., the frontal cortex) by analyzing the transmission and absorption of near-infrared light (700–950 nm) as it passes through tissue. Since biological materials, including skull bones, are transparent to this light spectrum, continuous non-invasive monitoring of brain oxygen supply is possible. Electrodes are adhered to the head, and monitoring begins with the induction of anesthesia (general, regional, or local). It is important to avoid hyperextension or extreme rotation of the head, which could compromise circulation.

If significant brain ischemia is detected, an intraluminal shunt should be applied to prevent neurological consequences. A relative drop of 15–20% in tissue oxygen saturation indicates critical brain ischemia. Additionally, stump pressure measurement after clamping the common and external carotid arteries can be used; a stump pressure of <40 mmHg suggests the need for an intraluminal shunt [5]. If the operation is performed under locoregional anesthesia, any new neurological symptoms observed during conversation with the patient necessitate the placement of an intraluminal shunt (Fig. 6.6).

There is no conclusive evidence that an intraluminal shunt should be routinely used during carotid endarterectomy. Therefore, it is advisable to use the shunt selectively based on the specific needs of the patient [6].

6.2.2 Arterial Reconstruction and Patch Angioplasty

If the artery's suture is longitudinal and the diameter is less than 4 mm, there is a risk of slight narrowing. Patch angioplasty helps prevent this issue. The patch is cut into an ellipsoidal shape and sutured with a running 6–0 polypropylene suture to close the arteriotomy.

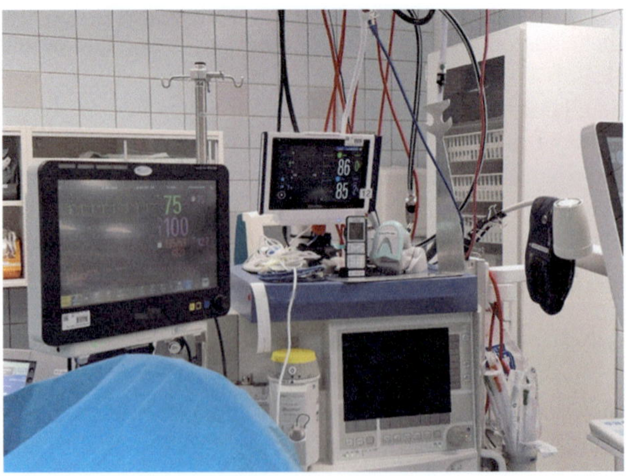

Fig. 6.5 Near-infrared cerebral spectrophotometry measurement should be taken before the surgery begins

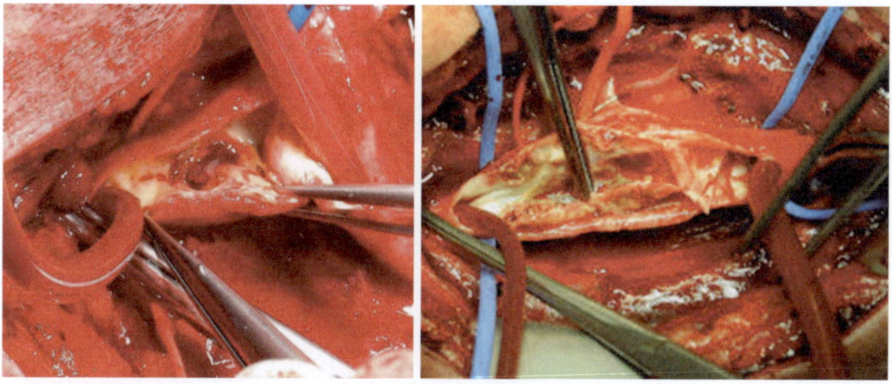

Fig. 6.6 Carotid endarterectomy with an intraluminal shunt

The materials used for the patch can include:

- Autologous vein (usually the saphenous vein or one of its branches).
- Autologous arteries (such as a segment of the external carotid artery or a portion of the cleaned occluded internal carotid artery after endarterectomy).
- Bovine pericardium.
- Synthetic materials, including polyester (Dacron) and polytetrafluoroethylene (PTFE). Note that PTFE can be prone to bleeding through suture points.

A suitable patch for angioplasty should always be longer than the endarterectomized segment. A well-tailored patch graft must not be too narrow, as this could compromise the prevention of stenosis at the suture line. When closing the artery with a patch, an intraluminal shunt, ideally placed before the endarterectomy, is necessary to minimize the duration of temporary brain ischemia. After reconstruction, circulation is first restored to the external carotid artery and then to the internal carotid artery. This sequence helps prevent possible microembolization to the brain.

6.3 Open Surgical Treatment of Symptomatic Carotid Stenosis with Eversion Endarterectomy Technique

Eversion carotid endarterectomy is a significantly improved variation of the classical procedure. It allows for complete cleaning of the carotid artery in a shorter time interval, eliminating the need for patch angioplasty and reducing stenosis risks (Fig. 6.7). Eversion carotid endarterectomy involves:

- Transection at the level of the carotid bifurcation.
- Removal of atherosclerotic plaque by twisting the artery.
- Anatomical reimplantation of the internal carotid artery.

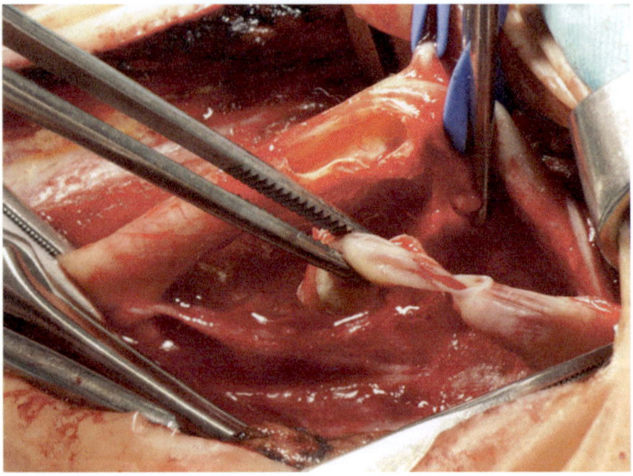

Fig. 6.7 Eversion carotid endarterectomy technique with plaque removal

Eversion endarterectomy is typically performed with ease, which helps reduce clamping time. The average clamping time is approximately 7–8 min.

Thrombendarterectomy involves the complete removal of atherosclerotic intima and media causing critical stenosis or occlusion of the artery. For successful endarterectomy, proper entry into the layer of the lamina elastica externa is crucial. If performed correctly, the procedure can be rapid, which is important given the artery's role in supplying the brain. Entering the appropriate layer, where the plaque is thickest or calcified, facilitates easier removal. After arteriotomy and flushing out the open artery's lumen, the atherosclerotic plaque typically separates from the external elastic lamina, which is the ideal layer for endarterectomy. The plaque is then removed, leaving a smooth surface without intimal leaflets or irregularities. Properly entering this layer ensures that a long segment of atherosclerotic intima and media is removed efficiently.

In cases of extensive plaque in the common carotid artery, particularly when it causes occlusion, Vollmar's semi-closed endarterectomy technique can be used. This method often makes it easier to remove plaque from the internal, common, and external carotid arteries and their first branches. Eversion endarterectomy is especially effective for solid, calcified plaques, as they tend to separate from the laminae elasticae external spontaneously (Fig. 6.8).

Special care is required at the distal end of the endarterectomy. The procedure must be completed without residual stenosis or irregularities that could create turbulence once blood flow is restored. Turbulence may lead to wall thrombus formation (acute thrombosis) and subsequent neointimal hyperplasia (restenosis).

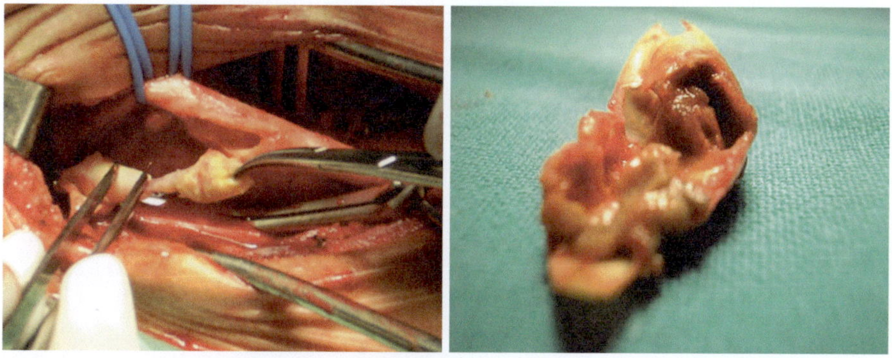

Fig. 6.8 Eversion carotid endarterectomy with plaque removal

Fig. 6.9 Reimplantation of the internal carotid artery using a Prolene 6-0 suture

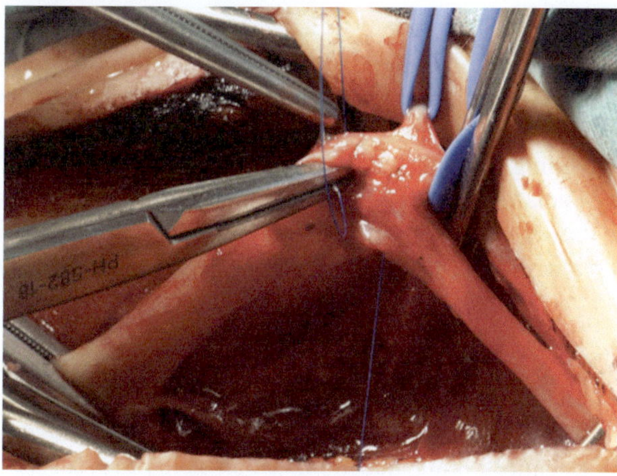

Eversion endarterectomy also allows for thorough examination of the ACI lumen, ensuring it is entirely clean, with no irregularities or internal flaps. Checking for retrograde flow from the ACI after endarterectomy is a standard part of the procedure.

6.3.1 Reimplantation of the Internal Carotid Artery

An extending, everting, non-absorbable Prolene 6-0 suture is usually used for sewing the artery. The operator always starts the suture from the farthest point, moving toward himself. The sutures must fall smoothly so that the edges of the internal and common carotid arteries are everted (way from the outside) so that the inside of the artery remains completely smooth without the eventual intrusion of remnants of the adventitia (Fig. 6.9).

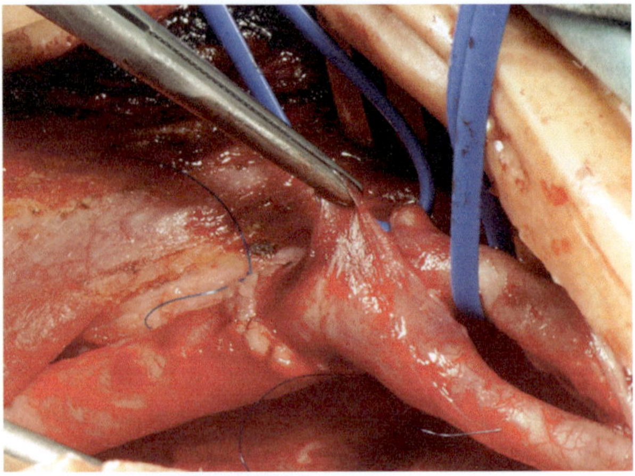

Fig. 6.10 Final results with complete vascular anastomosis and unclamped carotid arteries

Eversion carotid endarterectomy can be performed without error in less than 8 min, twice as long as traditional longitudinal endarterectomy (Fig. 6.10).

First, the clamp is removed from the internal carotid artery to flush out any remaining residue, and then the artery is reclamped. Next, circulation is restored to the unclamped external carotid artery. The common carotid artery is then unclamped to ensure that any potential microthrombi are directed into the external rather than the internal carotid artery. Finally, the internal carotid artery is unclamped.

6.3.2 The General Benefit of Cerebral Revascularization

- Proven to prevent stroke, reducing the risk by about 30 times during the first year.
- Enhances brain nutrition, which helps prevent vascular dementia and premature aging.
- Beneficially impacts the normalization of general, endocrinological, and metabolic status by normalizing pituitary gland function and the brain's neuroendocrine regulatory functions.

6.3.3 The Problem of Simultaneous Carotid and Coronary Disease

Atherosclerosis often affects both the carotid and coronary arteries simultaneously. In approximately 20% of patients who require coronary bypass surgery, there is also hemodynamically significant, albeit asymptomatic, carotid stenosis. Similarly, about 60% of patients undergoing carotid endarterectomy report symptoms of angina pectoris, and in 18% of these cases, coronary angiography confirms a significant degree of coronary artery disease [7]. If a patient requires both carotid and coronary reconstruction, the question arises: should the procedures be performed simultaneously or in stages? If staged operations are necessary, which procedure should take priority?

- Whenever possible, carotid and coronary revascularization should be performed with percutaneous angioplasty due to its lower risk.
- Patients with symptomatic carotid stenosis and stable coronary disease should first undergo carotid endarterectomy, followed by coronary bypass grafting after approximately 20 days.
- Patients with unstable coronary disease and asymptomatic carotid disease should first receive coronary bypass grafting. Carotid endarterectomy should not be delayed for more than 1 month, as this increases the risk of stroke.
- When necessary, patients with significant symptoms in both arterial systems may undergo simultaneous surgery.

6.4 Open Surgical Treatment of High-Grade Asymptomatic Carotid Stenosis

There is ongoing debate about the best treatment approach for asymptomatic patients with stenotic lesions at the carotid bifurcation, especially given the advancements in conservative medical therapy. In Scandinavian countries, a conservative approach for managing asymptomatic carotid artery stenosis has been practiced for an extended period. Additionally, some experts suggest that surgical intervention may not be necessary for most asymptomatic patients [8]. The necessity of revascularization is assessed on an individual basis, considering factors such as the degree of carotid stenosis, the morphology of the carotid plaque, the presence of comorbidities, and local anatomical characteristics.

European Society for Vascular Surgery guideline for average surgical risk patients with an asymptomatic 60–99% stenosis considers carotid endarterectomy in the presence of one or more imaging or clinical characteristics that may be associated with an increased risk of late stroke, provided 30-day stroke/death rate is ≤3% and patient life expectancy exceed 5 years [4].

Surgical treatment of asymptomatic carotid artery stenosis greater than 70% may be indicated if a silent brain infarction is documented on cross-sectional imaging. This is particularly relevant if another surgical procedure is planned soon, as certain plaque morphologies may increase the risk of perioperative stroke.

There is ongoing controversy regarding the benefits of carotid endarterectomy in patients with other carotid artery stenosis or occlusion, especially concerning long-term outcomes. In asymptomatic female patients, the overall benefit of endarterectomy is generally less than that observed in men.

For asymptomatic high-risk patients, angioplasty and carotid endarterectomy are not recommended if the operative risk exceeds 1%. In such cases, a conservative approach is considered the safer option.

6.5 Carotid Artery Kinking and Coiling- Treatment Options

Carotid artery kinking and coiling refer to the excessive elongation of the artery, which can occur due to an embryological abnormality or, in some cases, develop later in life due to factors like atherosclerosis and hypertension. Most patients are asymptomatic and do not require surgical treatment. In cases of incidental discovery, acetylsalicylic acid (aspirin) is often prescribed. Kinking and coiling can occur bilaterally and may be accompanied by atherosclerotic disease in the carotid artery. When these conditions cause hemodynamic problems and insufficient blood flow, they can lead to ischemic brain symptoms and discomfort, such as dizziness, fainting, and headaches, which may be exacerbated by head and neck movements [9].

There is no standardized criterion for color Doppler ultrasonography in assessing carotid artery coils and kinks. However, symptomatic patients with these conditions should undergo their first Doppler ultrasound examination. At the author's institution, symptomatic kinking and coiling of the carotid arteries are considered hemodynamically significant if the peak systolic velocity exceeds 200 cm/s (Figs. 6.11 and 6.12). Nevertheless, the ultrasound findings must always be confirmed by computed tomography (CT) angiography or magnetic resonance (MRI) angiography and correlated with clinical symptoms (Figs. 6.13 and 6.14).

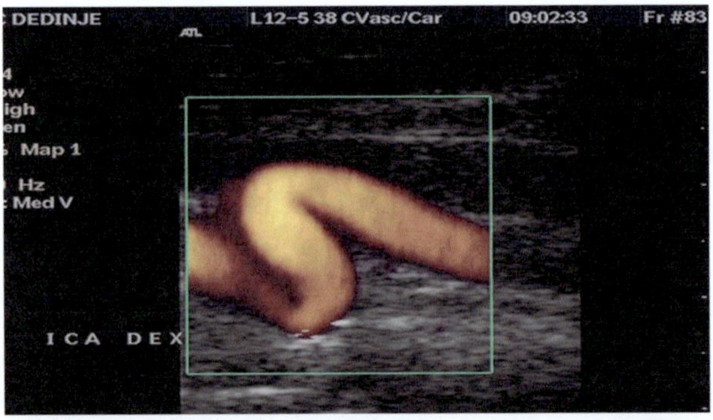

Fig. 6.11 Power Doppler ultrasound examination showing internal carotid artery kinking

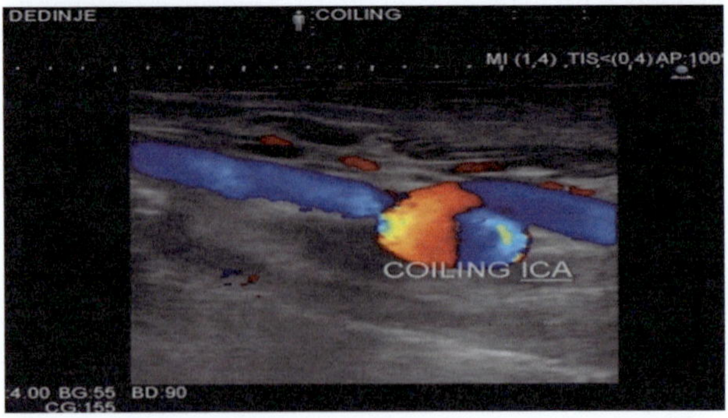

Fig. 6.12 Color Doppler ultrasound examination showing internal carotid artery coiling

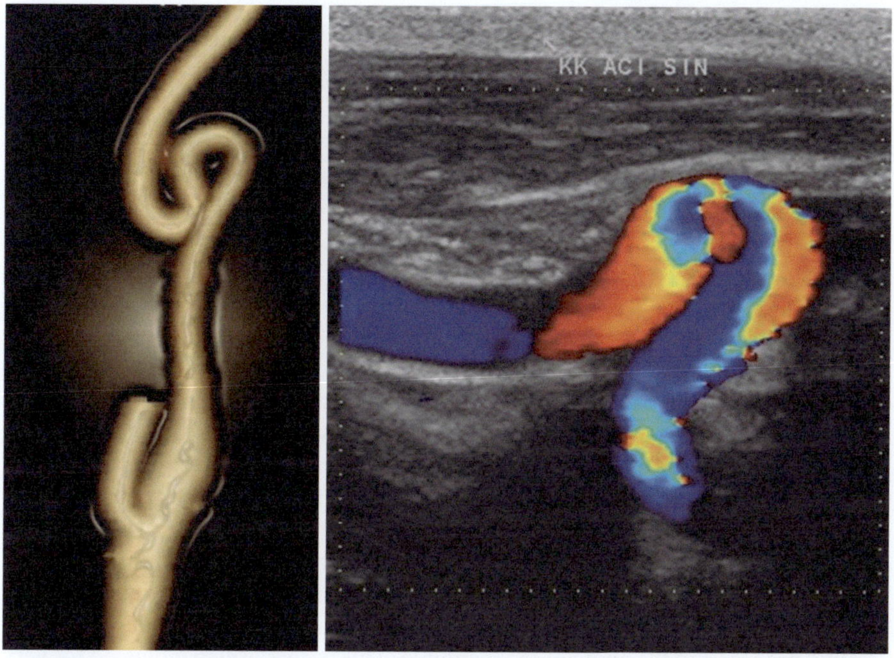

Fig. 6.13 Computed tomography reconstruction and color Doppler ultrasound showing internal carotid artery kinking

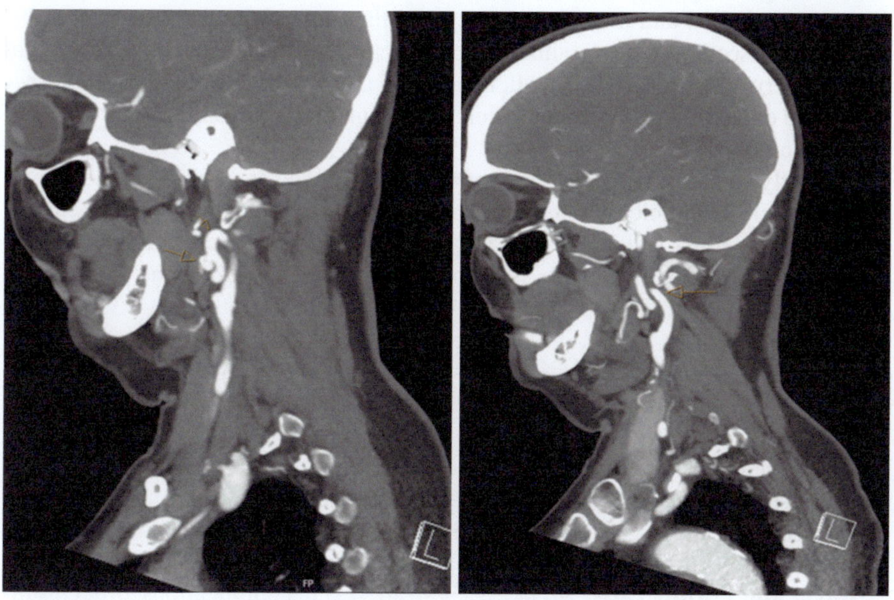

Fig. 6.14 Computed tomography sagittal reconstruction showing internal carotid artery kinking and small aneurysms (indicated by an arrow)

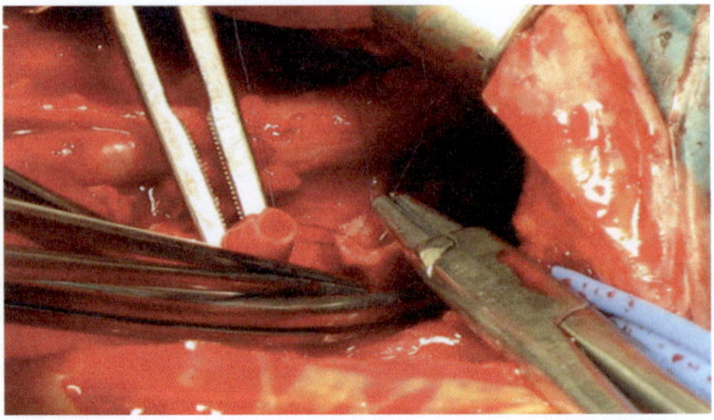

Fig. 6.15 Intraoperative findings showed carotid artery kinking, necessitating reconstruction and shortening of the artery

Surgical treatment of kinking and coiling is indicated in patients suffering from intermittent brain ischemia with focal (hemispheric) symptoms. This intervention is recommended if ultrasound and arteriography confirm significant kinking and coiling of the carotid artery, and brain CT or MRI has ruled out other diagnostically significant lesions in the brain and cerebral arteries.

High access to the carotid artery is often necessary, as the kinking or folding is usually located just below the base of the skull. To ensure a reliable operation, the internal carotid artery must be exposed above the line connecting the top of the mastoid process and the angle of the mandible. This access is also indicated for very high atherosclerotic or degenerative lesions and aneurysms of the internal carotid artery.

Two surgical approaches are used: the anterolateral approach (involving mandibular subluxation and muscle resection) and the posterolateral approach (involving muscle resection, with or without mastoidectomy). When accessing the internal carotid artery at the base of the skull, it is crucial that mobilization and partial resection of the digastric muscle do not result in damage to the surrounding cervical and autonomic nerves.

The early and long-term outcomes of resecting kinking and coiling of the carotid artery are very favorable, with minimal postoperative complaints, such as local tingling due to trauma to local nerves (e.g., ansa cervicalis). More importantly, the procedure effectively eliminates symptoms of cerebral ischemia and reduces the risk of stroke (Fig. 6.15).

6.6 Postoperative Carotid Surgery Complications

Carotid endarterectomy is one of the most commonly performed surgeries in the vascular field. The complications can be categorized into general and local, with the latter being specific to the surgery. Mortality and stroke, as major complications, should be less than 3% in asymptomatic patients and less than 6% in symptomatic patients [4, 10].

Intra- and Postoperative Strokes: These are severe complications, often resulting from technical failures during the operation. An intraoperative stroke occurs immediately after surgery and while the patient is still awake in the operating room.

Urgent exploration is required in these cases, where an intimal flap or thrombus formation is usually found to be the cause (Figs. 6.16, 6.17, and 6.18). If the stroke is due to intracranial thromboembolisms in smaller vessels, exploration may not resolve the issue.

Postoperative Stroke: This occurs after an initially uneventful recovery and is characterized by the emergence of new neurological deficits. Immediate computed tomography is indicated, and if necessary, neuroradiological thrombectomy may be performed (Figs. 6.19 and 6.20).

Hemodynamic Instability: Two-thirds of patients may experience hypertension, especially in the early postoperative period. This can lead to hyperperfusion syndrome, which may cause headaches and, in some cases, intracerebral bleeding (0.7–7.7%). Blood pressure control is managed primarily with labetalol (100 mg) or intravenous nitroprusside in complicated cases.

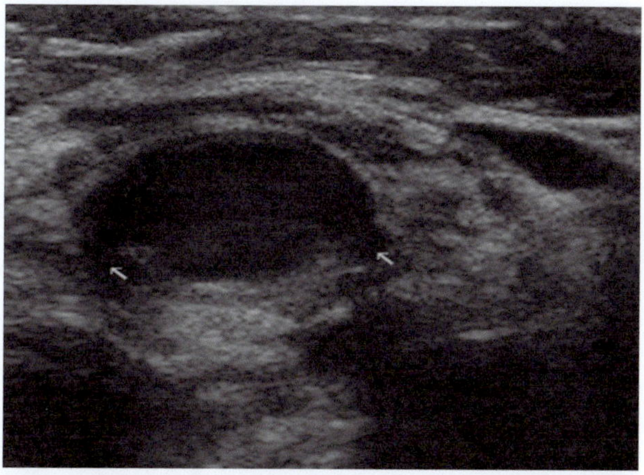

Fig. 6.16 Ultrasound examination showing postoperative acute carotid artery thrombosis

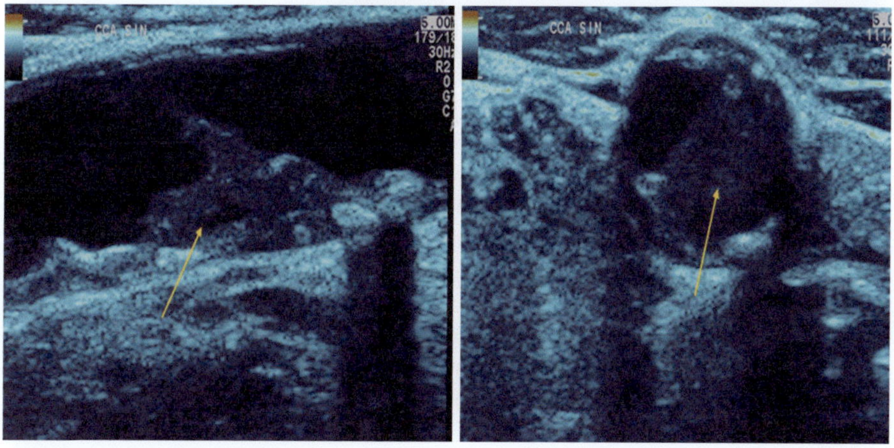

Fig. 6.17 Ultrasound examination showing a postoperative non-fixed intimal flap and partial carotid artery thrombosis (indicated by arrows)

Fig. 6.18 Ultrasound examination revealed a postoperative non-fixed intimal flap (indicated by an arrow) in an asymptomatic patient

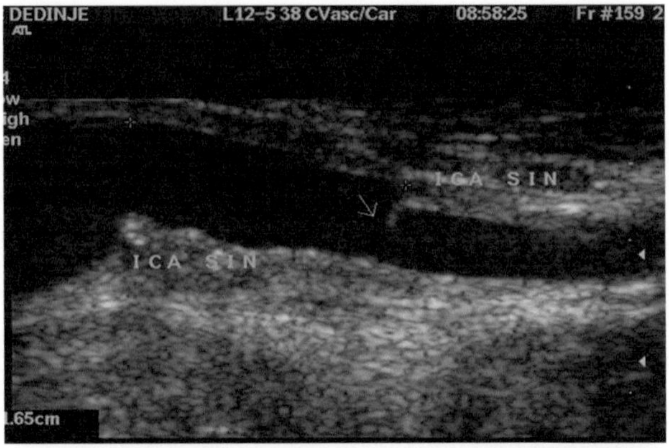

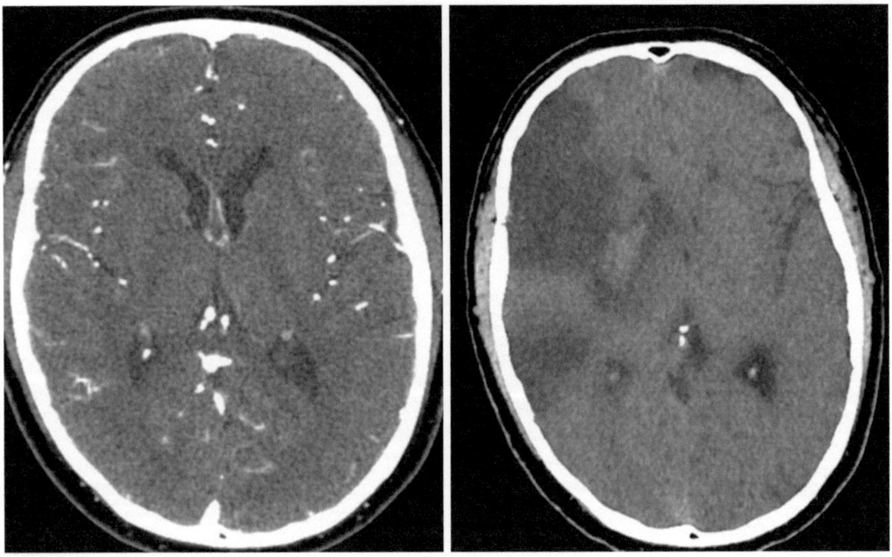

Fig. 6.19 Computed tomography before and after surgery revealed a massive postoperative stroke in the right hemisphere following carotid surgery

Postoperative Neck Hematoma: Occurring in 0.7–3% of cases, most neck hematomas are self-limiting. However, if the patient experiences pressure on the trachea and impaired respiration, emergency exploration is required (Fig. 6.21).

Nerve Lesions: These are usually temporary and can occur in 5–20% of cases. Affected nerves may include the marginal facial, posterior auricular, hypoglossal, laryngeal recurrent, and glossopharyngeal nerves.

Cardiological Complications: Primary myocardial infarction occurs in approximately 0.5–1.5% of cases.

Restenosis: This issue, due to neointimal hyperplasia or new atherosclerotic plaque formation, affects 5–22% of patients on long-term follow-up (Figs. 6.22 and

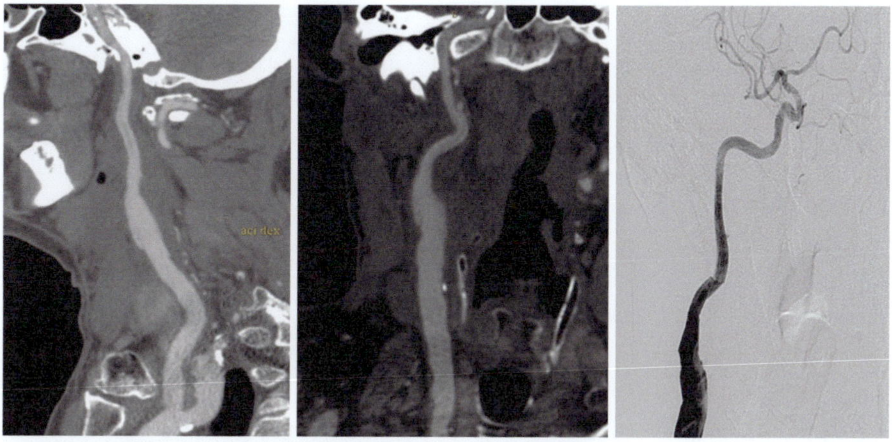

Fig. 6.20 Postoperative symptomatic carotid artery dissection identified on control computed tomography, and treatment with stent deployement

Fig. 6.21 Postoperative neck hematoma on the right side can be life-threatening and may, in some cases, require urgent intubation and exploration

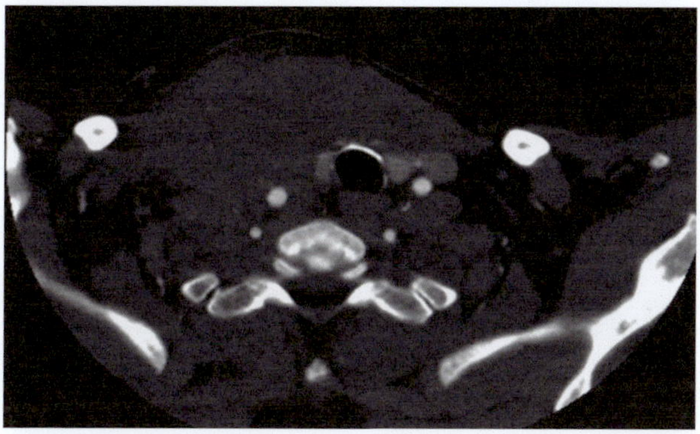

Fig. 6.22 Power Doppler ultrasound showing carotid artery restenosis after endarterectomy

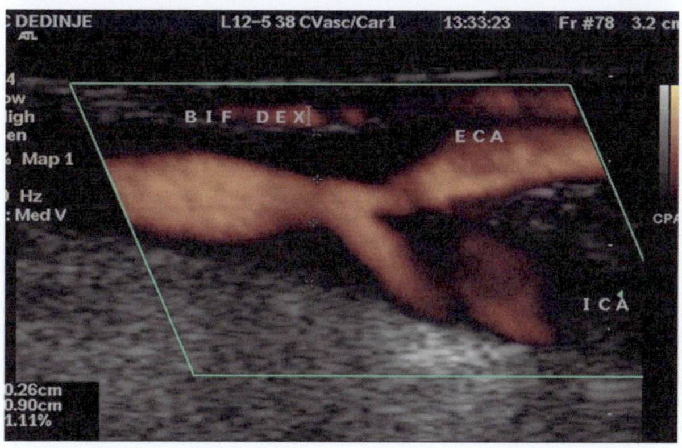

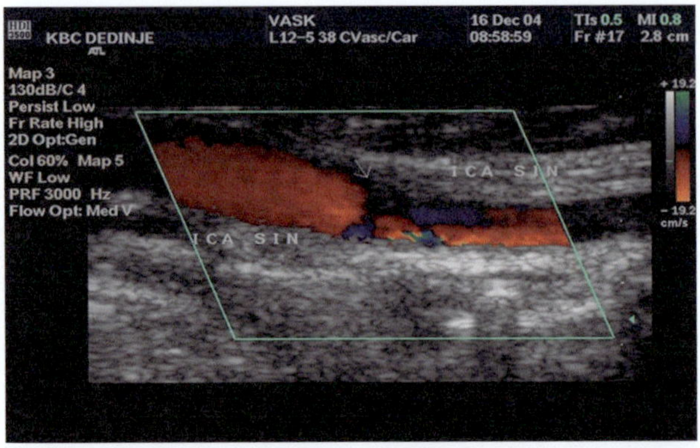

Fig. 6.23 Color Doppler ultrasound control showing carotid artery restenosis after endarterectomy

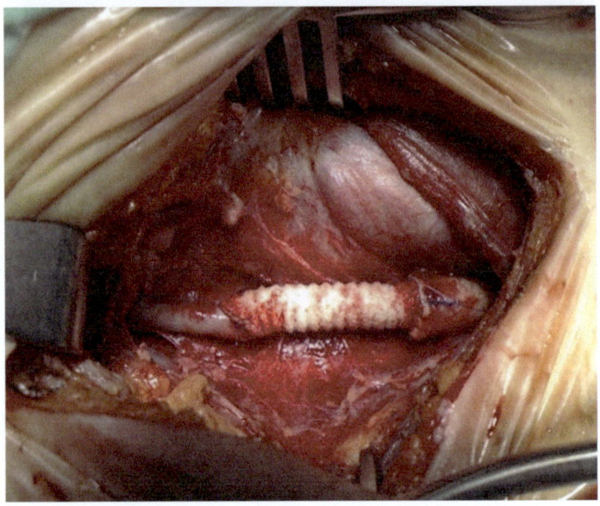

Fig. 6.24 Intraoperative findings after reoperation and carotid artery reconstruction with a vascular graft due to carotid artery stent thrombosis and recurrent ischemic symptoms

6.23). Symptomatic restenosis may require re-treatment, either endovascular or open surgery (Figs. 6.24, 6.25, and 6.26).

Infection and Pseudoaneurysm: These rare complications occur in 0.01–0.1% of cases and may present as abscess formation, fistulas, or pseudoaneurysms with bleeding (Fig. 6.27). The autologous vein is preferred for artery reconstruction, though ligation may be the only option in rare cases.

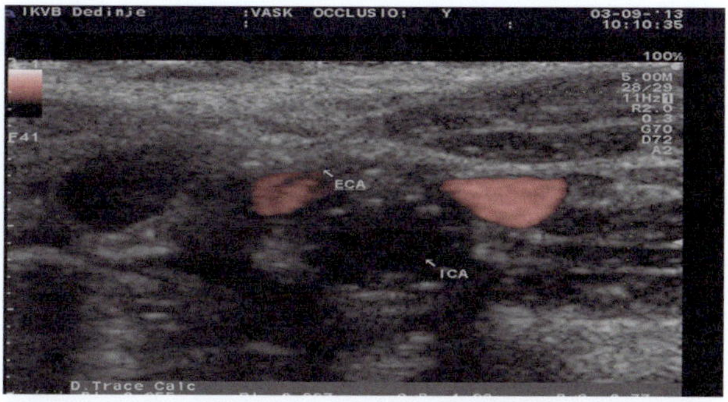

Fig. 6.25 Color Doppler ultrasound revealed complete thrombosis of the internal carotid artery stent

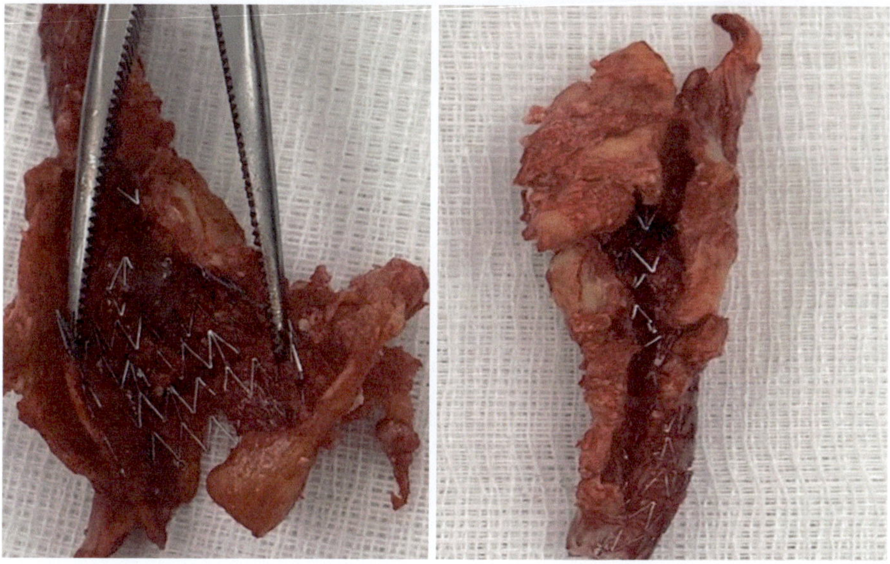

Fig. 6.26 Resection of the carotid artery, previously treated with a carotid stent and complicated by stent thrombus and fracture, was followed by reconstruction of the artery with a vascular graft

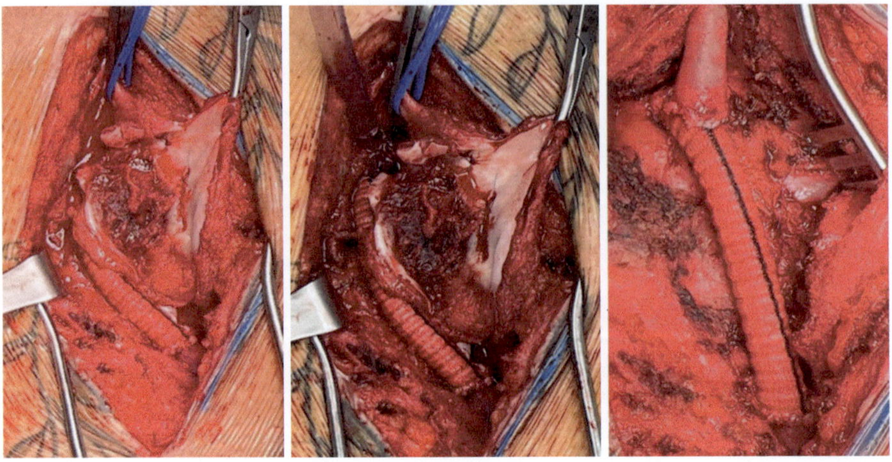

Fig. 6.27 An anastomotic non-infective pseudoaneurysm that developed after a previous carotid endarterectomy was treated with vascular graft reconstruction, external carotid artery reimplantation, and pseudoaneurysm resection

References

1. North American Symptomatic Carotid Endarterectomy Trial Collaborators. The beneficial effect of carotid endarterectomy in symptomatic patients with high-grade carotid stenosis. N Engl J Med. 1991;325:445–53.European Carotid Surgery Trialists' Collaborative Group. Randomised trial of endarterectomy for recently symptomatic carotid stenosis: final results of the MRC European carotid surgery trial (ECST). Lancet. 1998;351:1379–87.
2. Mayberg MR, Wilson SE, Yatsu F, Weiss DG, Messina L, Hershey LA, et al. Carotid endarterectomy and prevention of cerebral ischemia in symptomatic carotid stenosis. Veterans Affairs Cooperative Studies Program 309 Trialist Group. JAMA. 1991;266:3289–94.
3. Naylor R, Rantner B, Ancetti S, de Borst GJ, De Carlo M, Halliday A, et al. Editor's choice—European Society for Vascular Surgery (ESVS) 2023 Clinical Practice Guidelines on the Management of Atherosclerotic Carotid and Vertebral Artery Disease. Eur J Vasc Endovasc Surg. 2023;65:7–111.
4. Aburahma AF, Stone PA, Hass SM, Dean LS, Habib J, Keiffer T, et al. Prospective randomized routine versus selective shunting trial in carotid endarterectomy based on stump pressure. J Vasc Surg. 2010;51:1133–8.
5. Hommery-Boucher X, Fortin W, Beaudoin N, Blair JF, Stevens LM, Elkouri S. Safety of shunting strategies during carotid endarterectomy: a vascular quality initiative data analysis. Eur J Vasc Endovasc Surg. 2024;S1078-5884(24):00628–2. Epub ahead of print
6. Hao D, Jiang Y, Wang P, Mao L. A meta-analysis supporting the superiority of staged carotid artery stenting and coronary artery bypass grafting in patients with concurrent severe coronary and carotid artery stenosis. Medicine (Baltimore). 2024;103:e38665.
7. Naylor AR. Time to rethink management strategies in asymptomatic carotid artery disease. Nat Rev Cardiol. 2011;9(2):116–24. https://doi.org/10.1038/nrcardio.2011.151.
8. Desai B, Toole JF. Kinks, coils, and carotids: a review. Stroke. 1975;6:649–53.
9. Wu S, Wang H, Guo J, Zhang F, Pan D, Ning Y, et al. Comparative the effectiveness and safety of different carotid endarterectomy techniques: a single-center retrospective study. J Cardiothorac Surg. 2024;19:338.

Endovascular Treatment of Carotid Stenosis and Neuroradiological Thrombectomy

7

Goetz Benndorf

7.1 Introduction

Percutaneous transluminal angioplasty (PTA) and stenting of the (internal) carotid artery (CAS) for the endovascular treatment of carotid artery diseases have been introduced by a few early "brave men" like Klaus Mathias, Chuck Kerber, Jaques Theron, and Jiri Vitek in the early and mid-1980s [1–7]. Over the last 40 years, with numerous technical improvements in all aspects of the procedure including imaging, pre- and post-procedure medication as well as constantly improved tools and devices for stenting and embolic protection, the technique has significantly evolved.

Today, CAS represents a relatively well-established treatment choice for patients with significant carotid artery stenosis, especially for those who are at high risk for complications from traditional carotid endarterectomy (CEA). The development of modern stent designs such as dual-layer stents (DLS) and enhanced distal and proximal embolic protection devices (EPDs) has improved the safety and efficacy of the procedure [8]. Better selection of patients who are suitable candidates for CAS and increasing focus on preventing ischemic complications have improved the overall outcome. Currently, CAS is recommended for patients with symptomatic carotid artery stenosis (>50%) or asymptomatic stenosis (>80% or >70% depending on guidelines and patient characteristics). The decision often depends on the patient's surgical risk factors, associated comorbidities, and the individual anatomy.

G. Benndorf (✉)
Department of Radiology, Baylor College of Medicine, One Baylor Plaza, Houston, TX, USA
e-mail: benndorf@bcm.edu

D. Radak, S. Duvnjak (eds.), *Carotid Artery Disease: Surgical Perspectives*,
https://doi.org/10.1007/978-3-031-81842-4_7

7.2 Overview and Clinical Use of Tools and Devices for the Treatment of Carotid Artery Stenosis

Besides stents, balloons and other adjunct devices, diagnostic and guiding catheters as well as guidewires play a critical role in the performance of carotid artery stenting (CAS), providing access to the carotid artery and allowing for the navigation of stents and other devices during the procedure. Below is an overview of endovascular tools and devices commonly used for CAS.

7.2.1 Guidewires

The selection of appropriate guidewires (GWs) is vital for the successful execution of CAS procedures. As technology advances, newer guidewires with improved features, such as enhanced trackability and flexibility, are continually developed to optimize safety and efficacy for patients undergoing carotid interventions.

The majority of guidewires being nowadays used for CAS is hydrophilic coated to facilitate navigation while minimizing trauma to the intima. One of the most typical guidewires for basic supra-aortic access is the Terumo Glidewire® 0.035 (Terumo, Japan) that is in clinical use for more than 30 years and comes in a straight or a 45° J-shaped version. This guidewire is frequently used as the main access tool for diagnostic angiograms using 4-5F catheters as well as for placing larger 6–8 F guiding catheters. In tortuous, technically challenging anatomy, a slightly stiffer version that provides more support, is practical. Another useful Glidewire version with a shapeable tip has unfortunately become unavailable in Europe. It should be kept in mind that this guidewire must not be used to introduce a short femoral access sheath (11 or 23 cm) because withdrawal of such wire after puncture with 18G needle can cause coating damage and polymer shedding. Here, a standard teflon-coated J-wire, usually part of the introducer sheath packaging is recommended. The Glidewire is also available in 0.032″, 0.025″, and 0.018″ versions.

In cases where severely diseased, tortuous anatomy involving the iliac arteries and the abdominal aorta requires a more supportive system, the 150 cm 0.035 J-shaped Teflon-coated Emerald™ wire (Cordis Miami, Fl) is a widely preferred "workhorse" for femoral artery access. This wire also comes in 260 cm length, can be used for exchange maneuvers, and has 0.025 and 0.038″ versions, the latter being rarely needed nowadays. Stiffer wires, although sometimes helpful, carry a higher risk of vascular damage including vasospasm or dissection and therefore have to be used with great caution. Advancing even a standard 0.035 Glidewire into the petrous ICA portion should be done very gently under fluoroscopic control to avoid intimal injury. The typical armamentarium for CAS should include a number of guidewires with different lengths, tip angles, and stiffnesses.

For stent deployment, most devices come as monorail systems to be navigated over 0.014″ microguidewires (MGWs), among which the Traxcess® (Terumo-Neuro, US, Japan) and the Synchro2® (Stryker Neurovascular, Mountain View, CA) are very popular. For more support in challenging anatomy, stiffer wires such as the

Asahi Black (Asahi Chikai®, Intecc, Japan), ChoiCE PT Extra Support (Boston Scientific), and various 0.018″ wires are available. Most of them are hydrophilic coated and come as straight or pre-shaped versions. Newer promising developments such as the ARISTOTLE® (Scientific Vascular, UT, USA) have been introduced in the US.

7.2.2 Catheters

Constant evolution of catheter technology for CAS shows a clear trend "towards lower profile systems". Various angiographic catheters, typically available as 4-5F versions are available for diagnostic purposes and can, if of sufficient length (ideally >115 cm), also be used to place a coaxial or triaxial catheter system into the common carotid artery (CCA). Typical tip configurations for supra-aortic angiography are the Headhunter (100 cm 4F Supertorque™, Cordis, Miami, Fl) or the Multipurpose™ (MP, 125 cm, 5F Tempo®, Cordis, Miami, Fl) commonly used for right CCA/ICA access. Alternatively, a hockey stick configuration as found in the Berenstein catheter, available also in a 5F -130 cm version (Select® catheters, Penumbra, Alameda, CA), can be used to facilitate tracking of large guiding catheters.

For elongated arches, in particular, the left CCA in elderly patients with diseased and tortuous vessels, the Simmons (Sidewinder) 1–3 configurations are mainstay tools either in 4F or 5F (Supertorque™, Tempo™). These catheters are also provided by several other vendors in various diameters (4–7Fr). For CCA access with a coaxial or triaxial system, a 5F catheter (e.g., Multipurpose™ or Simmons-2 Tempo™) is the preferred choice. They are slightly stiffer than 4F catheters and usually tapered to 0.038″ guidewires providing more stability for placing large guiding catheters (or sheaths) such as the 80 or 90 cm NeuronMax® 0.88 (Penumbra) or the AXS Infinity® (Stryker Neurovascular, Mountain View, CA) as a suitable platform for stenting and thrombectomy (TE). Except for younger patients or relatively straight anatomy, a Simmons 2 ("Sim2") catheter is more or less a standard configuration for left CCA access during both diagnostic and interventional procedures. Penumbra offers the entire range of tip configurations as dedicated access catheters in sufficient lengths (120–130 cm) for selection and seamless transition with e.g., a NeuronMax 0.88 or the new Benchmark BMX 96 (inner lumen 0.096″) as well as any other guide catheter. They also accept 0.038 guidewires if more support is needed.

It must be emphasized that all catheters, especially guiding catheters and larger sheaths should be continuously flushed using pressurized heparinized saline bags to prevent (1) air-embolism and (2) clot formation with thromboembolism. The use of rotating hemostatic valves (RHVs, Y-connectors) and three-way stopcocks for that purpose is strongly recommended.

In general, large-bore guiding catheters, such as the NeuronMax 088, Infinity AXS, or the Super Arrow-Flex® sheath (Teleflex, Inc., NC) and others play a crucial role in CAS procedures as their proper selection greatly impacts the success and safety of the intervention. They provide access to the carotid artery, offer stability, and facilitate the introduction of balloons, stents, and other devices for embolic protection or thrombectomy (TE). The Infinity is currently offered as "Plus" version with 0.091″ inner lumen to accommodate the new Vecta74 (0.074″ inner diameter) for clot aspiration while maintaining an 8F outer luminal diameter.

Constant evolution of catheter technology for CAS shows a clear trend towards lower profile systems including 5F catheters for stenting. On the other hand, using larger systems for CCA access has the advantage that in case of an intraprocedural thromboembolism with, e.g., M1 occlusion, dedicated thrombectomy devices (TEDs) will require larger access systems to quickly reach and remove the clot.

7.2.3 Carotid Stents

Stents represent the most critical tool for the CAS procedure and have, since introduced, undergone multiple technical and design improvements. Several different types of carotid stents are currently on the market, each with specific features to optimize anatomic and clinical outcomes. They can be grouped according to their design (closed-cell vs. open-cell), material (bare metal vs. coated), shape (tapered vs. straight), and way of manufacturing (laser-cut vs. braided). Nowadays, more important is the differentiation into first generation, *single layer stents* (SLS) and second generation, *dual-layer stents* (DLS).

7.2.3.1 First-Generation (FDA Approved) Stents: Single-Layer Stents (SLS)

Closed-cell stent configurations:

- Xact™ (Abbott Vascular, Santa Clara, California)
- WallStent™ (Boston Scientific, Marlborough, Massachusetts)
- Scaffold™ (W. L. Gore & Associates, Flagstaff, Arizona)

Open-cell stents:

- Rx Acculink™ (Abbott Vascular)
- Precise™ (Cordis-Cardinal Health, Santa Clara, California)
- Protégé Rx™ (Medtronic, Minneapolis, Minnesota).

Mechanically, carotid stents are mostly self-expanding stents (vs. balloon-expanding peripheral or coronary stents) to optimally accommodate the patient's individual anatomy. Key requirement is high flexibility to adjust to the often tortuous and sometimes irregular morphology while providing sufficient scaffold and radial force to (1) main vessel patency, and (2) keep the atherosclerotic plaque material at the level of the arterial wall. To maximize anatomical adjustment, especially in curved carotid bifurcations, open-cell designs such as the Protégé™ (Medtronic) or the Precise™ (Cordis, Miami, Fl) stents have been introduced. While offering a higher radial force compared to the WallStent™, and thus giving more support, they come with the disadvantage of providing less protection against plaque protrusion and debris migration into the downstream territory.

The Carotid WallStent™ (CWS, Boston Scientific, Natick, MA), one of the oldest stent platforms, is a closed-cell design and widely implanted device (extensively used by the author). And although providing less radial force, this stent has demonstrated to prevent more debris from migrating into to the lumen due to its significantly smaller "free cell area." A downside of this stent is the limited longitudinal flexibility due to its braided tubular mesh design [9].

The Xact™ *Stent* (Abbot, Chicago, IL) is a newer closed-cell stent with a variable-cell design to offer "targeted" radial strength while minimizing plaque protrusion [10]. In general, closed-cell-design stents are inherently inferior in terms of accommodation to curved irregular anatomy and vessel wall apposition.

The AccuLink™ *or Xact*™ stents (Abbot) represent a different approach to improve accommodation to vascular morphology and specifically to the change in diameter between post-bifurcation ICA (often 4–5 mm) and the distal CCA lumen (usually 7–9 mm) [11]. The advantage here is that the smaller ICA lumen is less exposed to oversizing, and thus exposed to a lower chronic outward force that can lead to inflammation and restenosis [12].

Most currently available SLSs are bare metal, either laser-cut or braided and made of stainless steel, nickel-titanium alloy (nitinol), or cobalt-chromium-nickel Elgiloy (CWS). Stainless steel has a high radial force, an advantageous property to prevent device collapse but it is also more rigid, and thus may be associated with vessel wall injury, suboptimal wall apposition, and more inflammatory response leading to restenosis [13, 14]. Although cobalt alloys should have properties that allow better conformation to curved anatomy, restenosis has been reported as well [9, 15]. Nitinol, an alloy of nickel and titanium exhibits properties very suitable for self-expanding stents due to its shape memory and superelasticity combined with a low chronic outward force [12].

Among single-layer devices, the braided closed-cell Caresto®Stent (Acandis, Pforzheim. Germany) represents a novel development where the nitinol-platinum composite wire is treated with a special coating to reduce thrombogenicity. This so-called *Heal-Technology* consists of a covalently bound heparin coating to minimize the activation of platelets and coagulation cascade (to provide an "antithrombogenic-anti-inflammatory-endothelialisation-promoting" effect). This stent comes in sizes between 6 and 10 mm and is currently under clinical investigation.

7.2.3.2 Second-Generation Stents: Dual-Layer Stents (DLS)

- Casper™ aka RoadSaver™ (Terumo-Neuro, USA/Japan), not FDA approved
- C-Guard™ (InspireMD, Tel Aviv, Israel), currently seeking FDA approval
- Gore Carotid Stent®, GCS, (Gore & Associates, Flagstaff Arizona)

The discussion about the optimal stent type and which embolic protection device (EPD) to use remains a controversy [16]. The observation that even with a stringent use of EPDs, minor strokes are still observed post-deployment and likely caused by insufficient plaque coverage due to a relatively large pore size or cell size area, has triggered the development of a different stent design. Aiming to further minimize plaque protrusion and debris migration during and after CAS, dual-layer stents

(DLSs) consisting of an outer scaffold for stable positioning and an inner finer mesh (or vice versa) with a much smaller cell size were developed to reduce peri-interventional as well as secondary postinterventional thromboembolic events [17–26]. The basic concept is to combine the mechanical characteristics of an open-cell design to optimally accommodate to curved vascular anatomy with the properties of a closed-cell design to prevent debris migration.

The Casper™ RX Stent, identical to the "RoadSaver™", is a 5.2F system consisting of an outer nitinol scaffold and an inner nitinol micromesh. The stent showed initial promise in reducing periprocedural DWI lesions [27] and lower complication rates [28–30]. Bosiers et al. [29] found the stent a "safe and effective device for endovascular treatment of subjects at high risk for carotid endarterectomy" in 100 patients, and Kahlberg et al. [30] reported lesser event rates in symptomatic and vulnerable carotid plaques as compared to other carotid stents.

The same time, a significant number of acute clot formations and post-procedure occlusions have been reported [19, 26, 31–33] which appears to be in contrast with some reports using the RoadSaver for elective CAS in asymptomatic and symptomatic patients [22, 23]. The Clear-Road study observed a 4.2% ipsilateral stroke rate and a 7.5% restenosis rate after 1 year.

The C-Guard™, introduced in Europe in 2015, uses a slightly different design (Fig. 7.1) with an inner nitinol scaffold covered by an outer closed-cell *polyethylene terephthalate* mesh. This stent has a larger free cell size area (16.25 mm^2) of the nitinol frame than, for example, the WallStent (1.09 mm^2) or the Casper RX stent with 0.38 mm^2 [17, 18]. This in theory should increase its conformability while at the same time, the smaller pore size (165 vs. 375 μm) increases its efficacy to

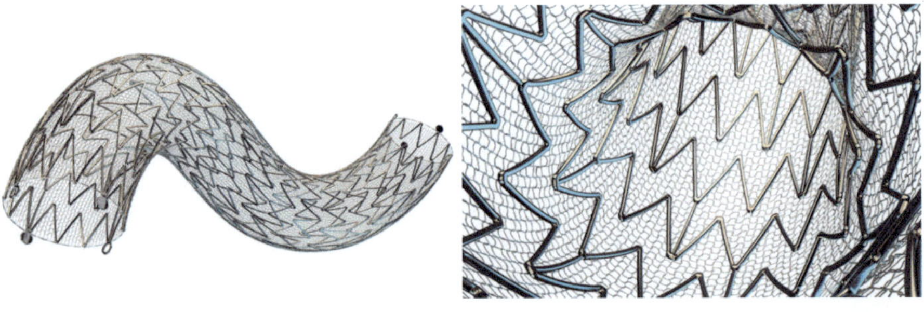

Fig. 7.1 C-Guard stent (Image courtesy Inspire, MD), dual layer stent (DLS). The C-Guard is a self-expanding stent made of two layers (second generation carotid stent). The inner layer consists of an open cell, nitinol laser-cut design. The outer layer consists of a MicroNet made of polyethylenterephthalat (PET) with small pore size (165 μm). This unique design combines the best of both worlds: open-cell design for optimal accommodation to curved anatomy and a micropore mesh to block plaque and debris protrusion, thus minimizes the risk of thrombembolism. Different from the Roadsaver (Casper) stent, the mesh layer to block debris migration is situated between the stent corpus and the vessel wall in direct contact with the plaque material. The stent is delivered via a rapid-exchange (monorail) system. The 6F delivery system is compatible with an 8F guiding catheter, the stent ranges from 6 to 10 mm diameter, 20–60 mm length and is advanced over a 0.014″ GW

prevent thromboembolism [34–36]. Results from several trials appear to support the concept of double-layer stents for both acute and elective CAS [17, 18, 36–40]. In two studies, patients undergoing emergent stenting for sub-occlusive stenoses and tandem occlusions showed a lower rate of stent occlusion when compared to single-layer WallStent [17, 18]. Klail et al., on the other hand, observed three cases of transient clot formation (9%) and one delayed occlusion in their retrospective series of 33 patients with acute ischemic strokes [39]. A review and meta-analysis of 17 patients found a ipsilateral stroke-death rate after 1 year of <1% and the pooled 1-year ipsilateral stroke-TIA/combined stroke-TIA rates were 1, 1.7 and 2.8%, respectively. The in-stent stenosis rate after 1 year was 0.8% [41].

When comparing the two commonly used DLS, the Casper™ RX (Road Saver™) and C-Guard™, it appears that the latter, although stent thrombosis may also occur [37], shows some superior performance. This is possibly be related to the different pore size of the micromesh (150–180 μm vs. 350–700 μm) and different construction with the protective layer on the outer side in direct contact with the vessel wall and thereby with the actual source of emboli [36, 41]. Obviously, more prospective data are needed to get an objective assessment and comparison of both stents and their future iterations [22].

Another interesting question will be, whether the use of DLSs in combination with proximal occlusion or flow reversal will eliminate the need for distal EPDs in the future. Considering that there will always be some patients who are not suitable candidates for ICA flow arrest, both techniques may be needed in the future and should be used complementary whenever required [42], (see below).

The GORE® Carotid Stent (GCS, W.L. Gore & Associates, Flagstaff, Arizona) is another DLS with hybrid concept incorporating both an open-cell outer part for optimal flexibility and conformability and an inner closed-cell portion consisting of an expanded PTFE lattice with a pore size of 500 μm to provide plaque stabilization [43]. It also comes with end-point covalently bonded heparin coating, the CBAS heparin surface. The first-in-man case was performed in 2013, and a recent study involving 312 patients showed 100% technical success and a low rate of periprocedural events and late strokes [44]. The stent is currently no longer offered by the company.

7.2.3.3 Other Stent Types

Covered Stents or Stent Grafts

These stents have a fabric cover attached to the metal lattice in order to prevent intimal hyperplasia (IH) and are used for longer, irregular stenoses and externally diseased arteries, e.g., chronic progressive stenoses due to post-radiation injuries or carotid blow-out syndromes [45–47]. Typical examples are the self-expanding Viabahn® Endoprothesis (Gore & Associates, Flagstaff Arizona, US), the Fluency® Plus Endovascular Stent Graft (Bard Medical, G, U), and the peripheral/coronary balloon-expanding Begraft® (Bentley InnoMed, Hechingen, Germany).

The Viabahn® Stent was FDA approved in 2005 and has been further improved since. The recent version has a heparin-coated expanded polytetrafluoroethylene (ePTFE) fiber mesh attached to an outer nitinol frame and is deployed by pulling a thread from a side hub. The stent yields clinical and patency benefits when compared to standard bypass grafts. It does require a 8–9F femoral access sheath for 5–7 mm target vessel diameter though and when deployed into a post-radiation necrosis tissue, infection is a serious risk. In a recent series of 24 patients with CBS undergoing treatment with both, Fluency and Viabahn stents, infections were observed in 16.7% [47]. Therefore, prophylactic administration of antibiotics should be considered. In addition, as with bare metal stents and despite heparin coating, strict DAP regimen and MP-testing testing prior to implantation (if elective) are as important as the post-deployment management (see Sect. 7.3.4). Acute stent thrombosis may be related to lacking patient compliance and discontinuation of medication whereas rebleeding may be prevented with monotherapy. Recently, the manufacturer offers also a balloon-expanding version.

The Begraft® (Bentley InnoMed, Hechingen, Germany), developed for peripheral and coronary vessels, combines a highly flexible one-layer stent graft with a low-profile balloon catheter and a small guiding catheter compatibility of 5F. About 100% of the CoCr stent surface is covered with a micro-porous ePTFE tubing of only 89 ± 25 μm. Experience in the supra-aortic and carotid arteries is still limited so far but device flexibility appears to allow navigation beyond the petrous ICA portion [48].

Biodegradable Stents

These stents have been in development for some time but have not made it to a clinically safe and feasible device yet. The concept here a device to provide temporary support which degrades over time, eliminating the need for long-term implant materials and related medication. While clinical trials are ongoing and data is not available yet, these stents may offer promise for reducing long-term complications associated with permanent implants and DAP medication [49, 50].

7.2.3.4 PTA Balloons

The use of percutaneous transluminal angioplasty (PTA) for carotid artery disease has preceded the implantation of stents [3] and is nowadays an integral part of both elective and emergent CAS. As with any other steno-occlusive disease, PTA has often to be performed prior to stenting (pre-dilatation) in order to gain sufficient luminal diameter, or after stent deployment (post-dilatation) to further improve the result. Numerous PTA balloon catheters have been developed and are in clinical use for peripheral and coronary arteries, many of which also feasible for CAS. In the author's clinical experience, the Maverick™ (Boston Scientific) is a very useful PTA balloon catheter that comes as a monorail system, tracks over a 0.014″ GW, and is available from 1.5 mm diameter in increasing 0.25 mm steps. For subtotal or even complete occlusion in emergent cases (e.g., acute complete occlusions), crossing the lesion using this smallest size low-profile balloon is often the initial step. In elective cases, subsequent stepwise dilatation under fluoroscopic monitoring using increasing pressure, and holding this pressure for 30 s to 1 min is usually preferred. The initial balloon size is typically based on the residual diameter but should also be chosen according to the planned end diameter of the artery in order to minimize the number of balloons and necessary exchanges during the procedure. A general recommendation is to slightly oversize the stent after PTA in order to achieve sufficient scaffolding and coverage of the lesion.

In emergent tandem occlusions, where a clot located more distally (M1) has to be removed as well, opening the severely stenosed or occluded portion just enough to allow crossing with an aspiration (intermediate) catheter is suggested (see Sect. 7.4). Then, this intermediate catheter is gently advanced into the distal or terminal ICA under repeated aspirations if clots are encountered here. Stenting is usually preferred after successful TE and not always needed as some highly stenotic lesions or occlusions will show a sufficient lumen after initial PTA and subsequent placement of a large-bore AC for extended period of time (dotter effect). Post-dilatation is required in cases with insufficient luminal diameter (<70%) due to rebound effect or lacking radial force of the stent.

However, although one rationale is to achieve full stent expansion and luminal gain while the risk of debris migration should be lower than with aggressive predilatation, great caution is advised. Especially with SLSs, post-dilatation should be in general minimized whenever possible, to prevent squeezing plaque material through the stent cells, and to avoid this so-called cheese-grater effect.

In acute CAS for tandem occlusions, no consensus exists whether to stent the ICA first and then remove the clot or vice versa. While both approaches have pros and cons, the majority of operators in the neurointerventional community would first perform intracranial TE to achieve as quickly as possible cerebral reperfusion. One additional argument is the observation that in some cases, the stenotic/occluded ICA lumen is sufficiently enlarged after initial PTA and added gradual "soft dilatation" ("dottering)" by the large GC.

One important aspect is to remember that any PTA in the ICA bifurcation may trigger periprocedural bradycardia and hypotension and requires the administration of vasopressors. This can be done either by selective atropine injection in patients who develop symptoms or as a prophylactic measure [51].

7.2.3.5 Embolic Protection Devices (EPDs)

With a constantly increasing number of CAS procedures being performed since the early 2000s, embolic protection has been considered a critical step to minimize the risk of stroke and other complications [52–55]. In addition to using sufficient intraprocedural anticoagulation, monitored activated clotting time (ACT, >250), and proper catheter flushing systems, this is mainly achieved by two factors: first, by the operator's skills and experience and second, by dedicated distal or proximal protection devices [16, 20, 53–65]. Only a few single center studies reported CAS without embolic protection devices [20, 66, 67]. Two main techniques of embolic protection have been developed and are currently in use [68–70]. Distal protection is achieved by deploying a particular device in form of a balloon or type of filter that stops and/or captures debris downstream from the treatment site. Proximal protection uses balloons for flow arrest, or flow reversal to prevent a priori the migration of embolic material by antegrade flow in the ICA [71–75].

While in the early era of EPDs, distal flow arrest using an occlusion balloon (PercuSurge Guardwire™, Medtronic) was mainly used [76], nowadays distal embolic protection is preferred and achieved using dedicated filters such as the Spider®FX (Medtronic) to not only capture but also remove debris that may be dislodged during the stenting procedure (Fig. 7.2). The use of distal (dEPDs) has significantly evolved, and their current state reflects advancements in technology, increased understanding of their clinical benefits, and evolving guidelines [53, 57, 65, 77, 78].

The following list shows some of the most commonly used devices and their pore size:

• FilterWireEZ® (Boston Scientific)	80–110 μm
• RXAccunet® (Abbott Vascular)	50 μm
• FiberNet® (Medtronic)	40 μm
• Emboshield® (Abbott Vascular)	140 μm
• SpiderFX® (Medtronic)	167–209 μm
• Angioguard XP® (Cordis)	100 μm
• Gore® embolic filter GEF (Gore & Associates)	

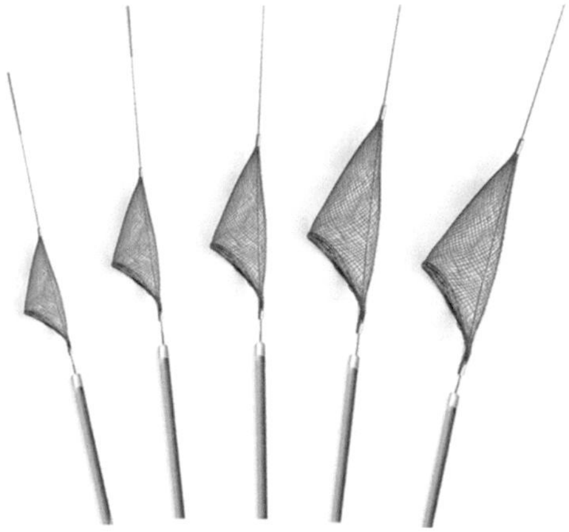

Fig. 7.2 Spider FX (Image courtesy Medtronic), distal embolic protection device (dEPD). This device was introduced in 2005 and consists of a braided nitinol filter that conforms to the vessel wall and should maintain full-wall apposition during the intervention. The idea is that blood flow is directed into the filter cone that will capture debris while maintaining flow in arteries (between 3 and 7 mm diameter). Although the nitinol ring helps to achieve circular wall apposition, in irregular and non-circular anatomy small gaps between device and vessel wall may allow some particles of debris to escape into the distal circulation. Other disadvantages of dEPDs are as follows: no protection during initial lesion crossing, protection limited by pore size, possible spasm, and dissection. Nowadays, a less frequently used EPD which can be delivered over a 0.014″ or 0.018″ guidewire

The SpiderFX® was introduced in 2007 and became a widely used filter for CAS. It is a braided nitinol design with independent longitudinal and rotational wire movement and a mouth indicator that provides enhanced visualization of filter opening. It can be used for lesion crossing using a 0.014 or 0.018″ and for target vessel diameter between 3 and 7 mm. This device was designed to contain and remove embolic material and is a distal filter that allows the operator to use the guidewire of their choice to cross the lesion and reach the target vessel portion.

Due to lacking data from randomized trials [79–81], controversy exists which technique, distal or proximal neuroprotection, is more effective. Both have pros and cons and require some operators' experience [64]. In inexperienced hands, a distal EPD (dEPD) carries a significant risk of complications by its placement alone including vasospasm, dissections, or even entrapment [60, 65, 82–84]. However, the main disadvantage of using a dEPD is the inherent risk of plaque dislodgement during the unavoidable initial crossing of the lesion [65]. No clear evidence exists that one filter device has benefit over another which suggests that operators should choose devices according to their level of comfort and confidence [16]. It must be noted though that no distal filter device provides 100% protection and embolic complications may occur regardless [85, 86]. Recently, Kim et al. reported a case of massive cerebral emboli despite the use of a distal filter [87]. Hong et al. recently described the occurrence of flow arrest in association with filter-type EPDs in 17.4% with a significantly higher rate of ischemic complications [60].

Some of these adverse events may be related to suboptimal wall apposition of the device [88] and particles of debris smaller than the micropores of the filter devices 100–150 μm [68, 69, 88–91]. A more recently trial-tested device, the Gore embolic filter (GEF, Gore & Associates) addresses some but not all of the inherent disadvantages of dEPDs. A diamond-shaped partial nitinol frame is circumferentially attached to ePTFE material with 100 μm pores and a hydrophilic heparin-bonded coating. The EMBOLDEN trial demonstrated safety and efficacy of this filter with a 1.2% major stroke risk and 3.6% rate of death or any stroke [16, 92].

The Neuroguard IEP® (Contego Medical, Raleigh, NC) developed to simplify the steps necessary to place a filter and to deploy the stent is another newer technology and consists of a "3 in 1 filter, carotid stent and post-dilation balloon system." The integrated distal micromesh filter with a pore size reduced to only 40 micron has been developed in part due to observations that a significant part of particle debris is actually smaller than 40 μm [93]. This device is currently under clinical investigation and was recently FDA approved. As a variant, the same manufacturer offers the post-dilatation balloon in combination with a filter as a separate device (*Paladin*, Contego Medical, Raleigh, NC) [94]. As recently pointed out by Chmiel et al., dEPDs like filters will continue to be associated with several inherent issues, including (1) unprotected crossing of the lesion, (2) potential filter or basket malapposition, (3) embolism by particles < filter pore size, and (4) limited filter basket capacity [85].

The alternative to a dEPD would be carotid occlusion using a proximal balloon (pEPD) which can be performed by creating flow arrest with or without flow reversal using the Mo.Ma™ (Medtronic) or the GoreFlowReversal (Gore & Associates) device [71–74, 95–98]. The Mo.Ma device, FDA approved in 2009, consists of a catheter carrying two balloons, one placed in the external carotid artery and another placed in the distal CCA (Fig. 7.3). The concept of this dual-balloon catheter is based on the fact that plaque material migrating into the ECA may also reach the cerebral circulation via ECA-ICA anastomoses [86]. The PROFI study showed a stroke rate of 2.3% while the combination of distal filter and proximal Mo.MA occlusion found a 30-day MACCE rate of 3.2% for filter use and 0% for the proximal occlusion demonstrating the efficacy of proximal protection [95]. This technique is, by avoiding lesion crossing prior to protection, conceptually more appealing than dEPDs [85]. However, it also comes with some disadvantages including a larger access sheath size and potential neurological intolerance of flow arrest in the ICA in patients with insufficient collaterals, a side-effect even seen sometimes during filter use [60]. In addition, the navigation of a balloon into the ECA as first procedural step, especially when stenosed, can be technically challenging and time-consuming in tortuous and severely diseased atherosclerotic vessels [98]. The device selection for embolic protection of CAS continues to be an ongoing debate. A meta-analysis comparing proximal and distal occlusion found no significant differences in terms of periprocedural stroke and 30-day mortality [81].

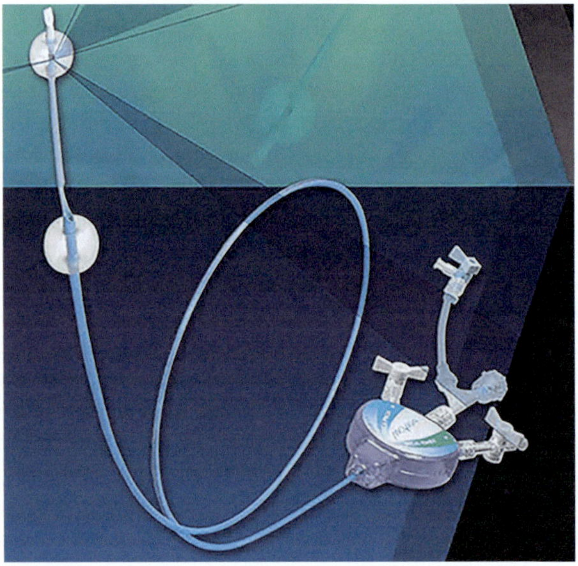

Fig. 7.3 Mo.Ma. Ultra (Image courtesy Medtronic, proximal embolic protection device (pEPD). An 8 or 9 F guiding catheter with an inner lumen of 0.069″ or 0.083″, respectively, and two highly compliant, elastomeric balloons to provide flow arrest and stability during CAS. The distal balloon is placed into the ECA and the proximal balloon into the CCA. For cases with occluded ECA, a one-balloon system is available. The system blocks antegrade flow in both ECA and CCA and allows flow reversal in the ICA by opening the sidearm for "backbleeding." The fundamental advantage over dEPDs is that embolic protection with MoMa is achieved "a priori," before the lesion is crossed with a guidewire. The combination of Mo.Ma. with DLSs is currently considered to offer the best neuroprotection during CAS

While the need of prospective trials is obvious, due to lacking Level 1 evidence, current guidelines are suggesting the use of EPDs for CAS at the discretion of the interventionist [99].

Real-world data from a large cohort study including 19.302 patients showed a generally low in-hospital risk of stroke [61] associated with the use of EPDs (proximal and distal). This study further demonstrated that the lowest risk of stroke is found in routine (1.8%) versus selective (2.9) or sporadic (3.1%) EPD centers. Therefore, some sort of EPD (proximal or distal) is currently recommended in Europe [61] and has become standard of care in the majority of US centers.

Furthermore, embolic protection using both, proximal occlusion with Mo.MA and distal filter has also been applied in a larger group of patients undergoing CAS using transradial and transbrachial access [42].

7.2.3.6 Transradial Access

Recently, an increasing number of patients undergoes CAS using transradial access (TRA). This alternative to the traditional transfemoral approach (TFA) has gained significant popularity in interventional cardiology. It offers certain advantages, especially in patients with advanced atherosclerotic diseases in the iliac arteries or abdominal aorta as well in cases with Type 3 aortic arches. Whether or not TRA will replace TFA in the future remains an open question for the time being. This approach has also its appeal for neuroendovascular procedures, especially in patients with challenging aortic arch anatomy or severe peripheral steno-occlusive disease but also in general for the patients' comfort. On the other hand, TRA has some inherent limitations [42, 100, 101], the most important one being the size of the radial artery (RA) with an average diameter in adults of 2.6 mm [102]. Therefore, this artery cannot easily tolerate large-bore guiding systems the same way as CCA and ICA do (usually 9–6 mm) and the introduction of 7–8F sheaths may become problematic, especially in female patients (RA = 2.2 mm). Although perceived in the beginning (2018–2019) by some neurointerventionists with great enthusiasm, until today, TRA has not replaced TFA and is mainly used for outpatients and FU studies. Because basic principles of catheter navigation, stenting, the use of EPDs and TE devices do not differ much from TFA, this section is kept short.

7.3 Overview and Clinical Use of Thrombectomy Devices (TEDs)

Acute ischemic stroke secondary to acute thromboembolic occlusion of the stented ICA or in the downstream circulation during or after ICA stenting is one of the most feared complications of CAS and requires immediate recognition and action [16]. The main goal is to restore blood flow as quickly as possible to prevent brain tissue damage and adverse neurological outcomes.

TEDs are important in the setting of elective CAS, when emergent thrombectomy (TE) becomes necessary as a bail out, or in combination with acute stenting of ICA occlusions often encountered as tandem lesions [103–105].

In 2015–2016, several major randomized trials (MR CLEAN, ESCAPE, REVASCAT, SWIFT PRIME, THRACE and EXTEND IA) [103, 105–109] demonstrated a clear benefit for stroke patients undergoing TE. Thus, the number of patients with AIS treated by mechanical TE has dramatically increased with indications constantly widening [104, 109–113]. As a consequence, thrombectomy devices (TEDs) have nowadays become a vital tool in treating acute ischemic strokes, especially in patients with large vessel occlusions (LVO). They are available either as stent retrievers (SRs) or aspiration catheters (ACs). In the setting of acute or elective CAS, knowledge, experience and skills to perform mechanical TE can be crucial to allow successful rescue of a thromboembolic complication and to ensure best possible clinical outcome.

7.3.1 Stent Retrievers (SRs)

Stent- or clot retrievers are advanced via a microcatheter and placed within the clot to (1) expand and engage, and (2) capture and remove the thrombus. Once the stent fully engages the thrombus (ideally after waiting for 1–2 min), the microcatheter (MC) and stent retriever (SR) are slowly withdrawn in order to remove the clot from the artery [108].

The first important step consists of navigating the MC through the clot over a 0.012″ or 0.014 microguidewire (MGW), e.g., a Traxcess™ (Terumo-Neuro, U.S./Japan) or a Synchro™ (Stryker). Typically, the MC is then placed slightly distal to the presumed distal end of the thrombus in order to deploy the stent retriever by unsheathing. Because the wire has to first cross the clot, followed by the MC, this maneuver carries the inherent risk of dislodging small thrombi or the entire clot into the downstream circulation even with simultaneous blockage of the flow by a proximally inflated balloon (flow arrest). As this step is unavoidable for any current mechanical clot retrieval device, additional simultaneous aspiration is recommended and minimizes the risk of untoward clot migration during the TE procedure (see below). Among a wide range of available devices, some currently popular and widely used SRs are the Solitaire FX™ (Medtronic, Irvine, CA) [114–122], the Trevo NXT™ (Stryker, Kalamazoo, MI) [116, 123–130], and the Embotrap III™ (Cerenovus, J&J, Irvine, CA) [131–136] available in various diameters between 3 and 6 mm and lengths between 20 and 45 mm. Table 7.1 gives an overview of some SRs and their dimensions.

Table 7.1 Dimensions (diameter and length) of three popular and widely used SRs in mm

Trevo NXT		EmbotrapIII		SolitaireX	
3	32	5	22	3	20/40
4	28	5	37	4	20/40
4	41	6.5	45	6	24/40
6	37				

Stent Retrievers (SRs)

- Solitaire™ (Medtronic)
- Embotrap™ (Cerenovus)
- Trevo™ (Stryker)
- CatchView™ Mini (Balt)
- pREset™ (Phenox)
- Tigertriever™ (Rapid Mecial)
- CascadeNet™ (Perflow Medical)
- Eric® (Terumo-Neuro, US/Japan)
- NeVa™ (Vesalio)
- Mindframe™ (Medtronic)
- Revive™ (Codman Neuro/DePuy)
- 3D Revascularization Device™ (Penumbra)
- Aperi® (Acandis)

After the *Merci Device*, the first dedicated clot retrieval device introduced in 2004 [137], the *Solitaire* was the next widely used SR. Its design was originally based on a stent developed for stent-assisted coiling of wide neck aneurysms, and the first clot retrieval was performed in 2008 [138]. It is a non-circular hollow tube nitinol structure with a closed-cell scaffolding design and longitudinal overlap that allows to accommodate arteries of varying diameter. Besides the REVASCAT study in 2015, the stent has been used in multiple clinical trials [108, 114, 115, 117, 119, 121, 122, 139–141].

The Trevo NXT is a newer, 3rd-generation thrombectomy device that was clinically investigated in its initial design in 2010–2011, followed by multiple subsequent trials [123, 125, 127, 128, 130, 138, 141–149]. The current version has "TriGlide" delivery wire that should facilitate a smoother and easier delivery and withdrawal into the aspiration catheter for "hybrid-thrombectomy" (Fig. 7.4). While the Trevo's radial force is similar to the Solitaire, its distal tip is slightly tapered and its fluoroscopic visibility better due to implemented platinum wires. Some studies showed superior performance with higher successful recanalization rate, shorter procedure time, lower number of passages, and better first pass rate compared to Solitaire [128].

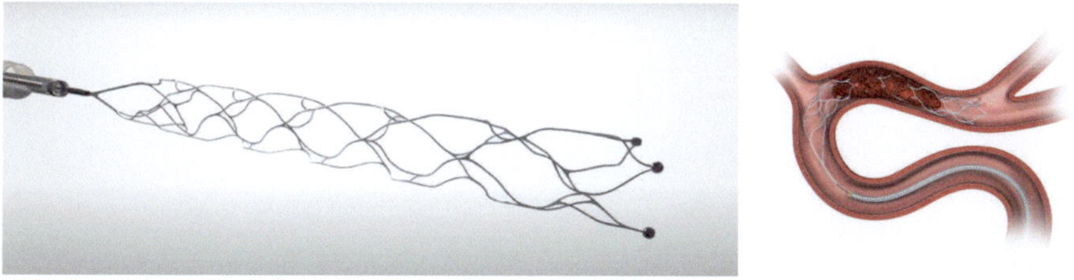

Fig. 7.4 Trevo NXT (Image courtesy Stryker). Popular tubular stent retriever with good visibility, advanced via 0.021″ MC (e.g., TrevoTrak21, Rebar). To avoid friction, it is important to sufficiently wet the stent retriever in saline prior to introduction into the MC. Frequently used by the author for M1 and M2 occlusions

The Embotrap III, introduced in 2015–2016 [131, 150], is another a 3rd-generation SR with "3-dimensional" design aiming not only to catch but also to hold on to the clot better, and thereby lower the risk of clot fragmentation and distal embolization [150]. It consists of a nitinol-made inner tube structure with outer cages where the distal mesh (cage) has now a smaller cell size than previous versions (Fig. 7.5). This last cage is tapered distally, the others proximally to minimize trauma during deployment and retrieval. Added iridium-platinum wires offer good radiographic visibility which is important to monitor deployment and the degree of engagement with the clot. The Embotrap comes in 5 and 6.5 mm only (see Table 7.1) and has been evaluated in multiple trials [116, 133–136, 151–155]. It has been used extensively by the author as an alternative to the Trevo. Considering the large and ever-increasing number of clot retrieval devices, it has become difficult to evaluate and realistically compare different stent retrievers in terms of their technical performance and achieved clinical results. In the author's experience, it appears reasonable to have more than one type of SR on the shelve in order to switch should one device fail and the next one (and sometimes inexplicably) would work.

Microcatheters used for SRs between 4 and 6 mm diameter (M1 occlusions) are usually 0.021″ catheters, such as Rebar™18 (Medtronic) with 160 cm length and a 2.4F distal OD or the TrevoTrak™ (Stryker) with 162 cm length and a distal OD of 2.4 F.

In a normal sized MCA (M1 = 2.6 mm), a 6 mm device should be attempted first. Although claimed otherwise by industry as well as some operators, technical differences between various types of currently available SRs and their efficacy are more or less marginal and appear to have little or no influence on the success rate or the clinical outcome [116, 140]. A meta-analysis (MASTRO1) found that EmboTrap may be associated with improved functional outcomes when compared with Solitaire and Trevo. On the other hand, EmboTrap and Trevo were associated with lower rates of

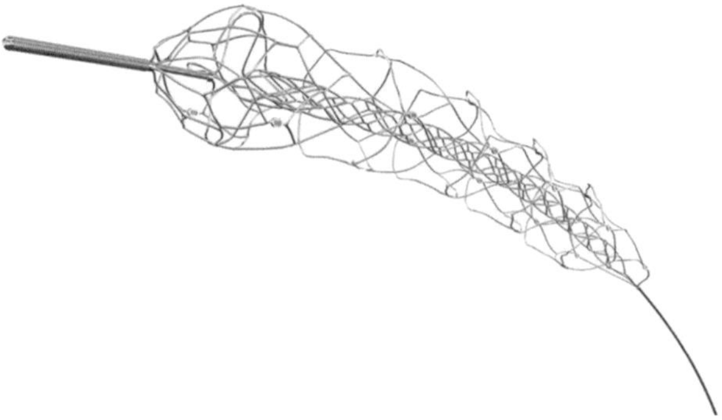

Fig. 7.5 Embotrap III (Image courtesy Cerenovus): Stent retriever with a more complex 3D design (inner tubular and outer cage structure) with good visibility, advanced via 0.021″ MC (e.g., Rebar18, TrevoTrak21). Improved third generation with denser mesh of distal cage. Utilized by the author as alternative to Trevo in cases with "difficult to retrieve" clots

intracranial hemorrhages (ICH) and mortality compared with the Solitaire. However, no significant differences in recanalization and thromboembolism in new territories were found and results were considered heavily confounded by various factors such as variations in thrombectomy techniques which highlights the need for RCTs to obtain Level 1 evidence [116].

During SR pull-back, simultaneous aspiration should be applied to the guiding (coaxial system) or better the intermediate (aspiration) catheter (triaxial system), either manually using a vacuum syringe (Vaclok®, Merit Medical) [156] or with a dedicated aspiration pump ("hybrid thrombectomy") [126]. For more distal occlusions (M 2–4 segments), a 0.017″ MC, e.g., the HEADWAY™17 (Terumo-Neuro, US, Japan) or smaller MCs can be navigated over a 0.014 GW to deploy smaller retrievers (3–4 mm). Caution is needed when approaching cerebral vessels beyond the M1 segment as distal cerebral arteries are more fragile and prone to dissection and perforation during advancement and manipulation of wires, catheters and during the retrieval of thrombus using metal stents. Therefore, tips of MGWs should be shaped into a a small "double-J" or "loop" to minimize vessel trauma and facilitate advancement through narrowed and thrombosed vessels ("loop technique") [157].

The Tigertriever™ (Rapid Medical, Israel) is a newer, different type of clot retrieval device based on the Comaneci device, a fine mesh that was developed for treatment (remodeling) of wide-necked cerebral aneurysms (Fig. 7.6). The Tigertriever comes as XL, 17 and 13 version (0.021″, 0.017″, 0.013″) with the Tigertriever™13 being particularly interesting for very distal occlusions 0.013″ MCs (1.3 F, Terumo-Neuro, U.S./Japan) [158, 159]. The unique feature of this device is the proximal and distal tapering as well as the gradually (by small increments) controllable deployment mechanism that is easy to monitor due to the high

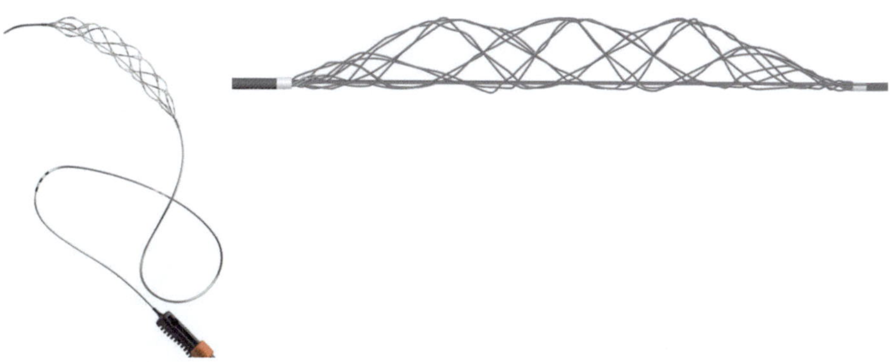

Fig. 7.6 Tigertriever (Image courtesy Rapid Medical). Stent retriever based on the Comaneci device with a tapered proximal and distal end, available as Tigertriever XL (21), 17 and 13. The Tiger13 is the lowest profile SR currently available and compatible with a 1.3F microcatheter (HeadwayDuo 167 cm, TerumoNeuro) for very distal occlusions. Another unique feature is the click mechanism that allows to gradually expand and collapse the device which is well visible under fluoroscopy due to its high radiopacity. While the device is highly flexible and vessel compliant, it does tend to create a banana-shape when fully opened in small arteries. Successfully used by the author for M3-M4 occlusions

radiopacity. Compared to the other SRs, it is relatively smooth to deploy and retrieve from M3 and even M4 branches without significant spasm or a high risk of dissection (author's experience). The device has been evaluated in a number of studies [160–165]. In a recent analysis of literature data, the Tigertriever13 performed similar to other devices regarding reperfusion rates in distal medium vessel occlusions [158].

7.3.2 Aspiration Catheters (ACs)

These catheters use simple suction, either applied manually using a vacuum-lock syringe or via a vacuum pump to directly remove the clot from the vessel. This technique can be particularly fast and efficient with clots that are soft, located in straight vessel segments (e.g., M1) and fully occlusive. The concept of direct aspiration first pass effect technique (ADAPT) was introduced in 2014 [166] and has been adopted since by many operators mainly because of its simplicity and efficacy when compared to the use of a retrieval device. Most major vendors now offer aspiration catheters between 4 and 7 F with increasing inner diameters ("large-bore" or "superbore" catheters), however with minor differences in terms of their aspiration efficacy. Typical aspiration catheters are the new "RED™" family (Penumbra) [167], the CAT™ 5–7 series (Stryker), and the REACT™ catheters [168–170] from Medtronic (Fig. 7.7 and 7.8). Although primarily not developed for clot aspiration, the 5F SOFIA™ and 6F SOFIA™ Plus catheters (Terumo-Neuro, U.S./Japan) [171–184] have also gained large popularity, especially due to their excellent navigability (Fig. 7.9).

The original platform for mechanical thrombectomy using aspiration [185] introduced by Penumbra (ACE catheters) included also smaller catheters for distal clot

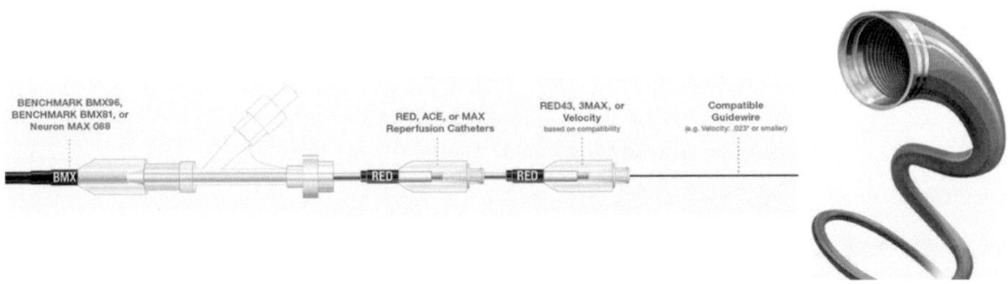

Fig. 7.7 Triaxial catheter system for aspiration TE (Image courtesy Penumbra) BMX96, 81 main guiding catheters with RED72 and 3MAX or RED 43 catheters. The original ACE series of initially developed ACs from Penumbra has recently been replaced by the "RED" catheters with new outer lining and improved trackability. Added smaller diameter catheters like the RED 43 and 4MAX complement the series to go further distal and perform aspiration TEs in M2-M3 branches. At the same time, the length of 3MAX and RED43 (160 cm) allow easier distal navigation of the large-bore versions (RED72 and 68) into the M1. All ACs developed and manufactured by Penumbra are intended for direct clot aspiration (ADAPT) rather than as intermediate catheters and are reinforced preventing catheter collapse during pump aspiration. The RED72 and RED 68 have been frequently used by the author

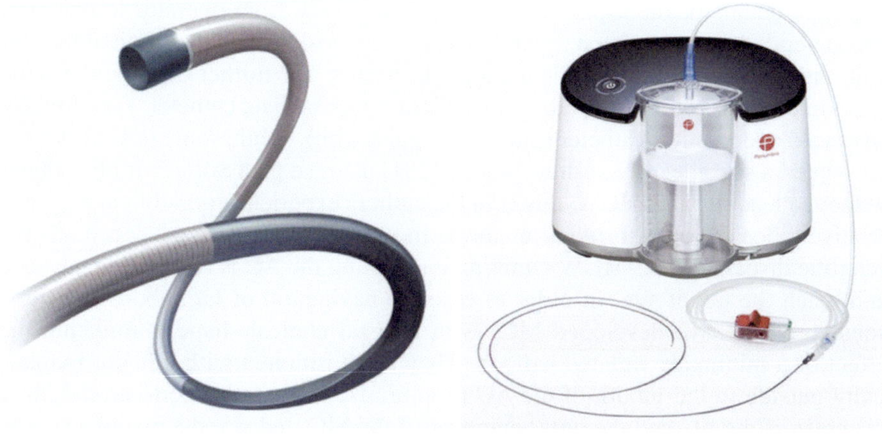

Fig. 7.8 Benchmark BMX96 (Image courtesy Penumbra). The new BMX 96 is an 8F guiding catheter that offers a larger inner diameter of 0.096″ and accepts the new RED78 with an inner lumen of 0.078″. The RED43 has the so-called REDGlide technology over its entire length (working length 153 cm) and a distal outer diameter of 1.5 mm which allows easier distal navigation and clot aspiration in M2-M3 branches. Compared to the 3MAX it has a slightly larger distal diameter but also an optimized lumen occupation (e.g., 83% vs 69% with RED72). The Jet Engine has been optimized and offers currently the most powerful aspiration force (vacuum: −29.2 in Hg) when used with the Penumbra reinforced tubing. The latter is important because non-dedicated (softer) tubings may, although more affordable, not provide full vacuum transmission to the AC tip, and thus reduce the effective aspiration force. The Penumbra tubing can also be used with any other AC (Sofia, REACT, etc.) and is the preferred choice of the author

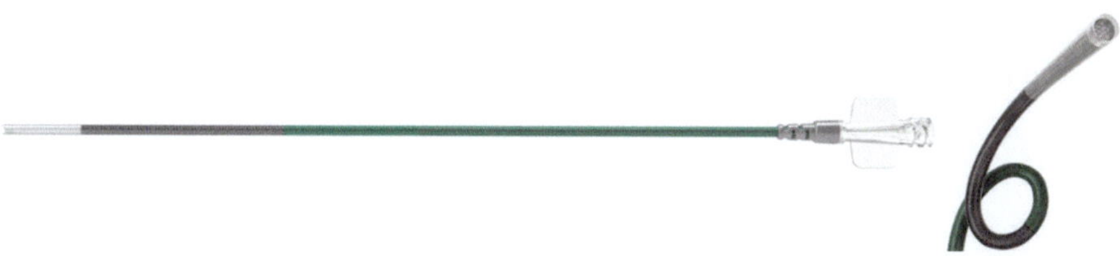

Fig. 7.9 SofiaPlus (Image courtesy TerumoNeuro). The 6F aspiration (intermediate) catheters in 125 cm and 131 cm lengths are also available in 5F and recently as a Sofia 45. This catheter with an inner lumen of 0.071″ was not primarily developed for clot aspiration but as an intermediate catheter for tri-axial catheter systems. However, its superior performance in trackability, in some cases even without a leading guidewire or MC (co-axial) has resulted in a wider acceptance as primary aspiration catheter. Its distal end is not reinforced and should be watched under fluoroscopy during stent retrieval as it can get damaged. Catheter collapse during pump aspiration has been reported and discussed as possible concern by some investigators, however remains overall a rare observation (not encountered by the author). The 6F catheter is very popular for M1 occlusions and also a good option for acute intra-stent clot formations in the ICA

locations (M2-M3, BA, PCA) such as the 5Maxx™ and 3Maxx™ catheters. Recently, the new RED43 for more distal aspiration of M2-M3 clots has been added to the portfolio as well. This trend is followed by other vendors, with the Sofia™ 45 (Terumo-Neuro) now available to further expand and apply the ADAPT technique to distal cerebral territories. In addition, Penumbra has launched a larger main GC, the 8F BMX96™ with an inner lumen of meanwhile 0.96 mm (Fig. 7.8).

While details of the aspiration technique may vary from operator to operator, one general concept has been so far, to engage the most proximal portion of the clot with the mouth of the AC while avoiding to push it any further distal at the same time. In order to achieve this goal, the AC (or "intermediate catheter") is carefully advanced over a microcatheter (plus micro guidewire). While some operators have advocated a so-called Snake-It technique [181] using, e.g., a Sofia 5 or 6F catheter without a leading MC-MGW, this is in the authors experience possible mainly in a relatively healthy, non-tortuous anatomy. In most patients with advanced athero-sclerotic disease, a MC-MGW combination leading the AC is required to advance and reach the target site. In order to ease the navigation of large-bore catheters, some vendors have developed MCs with a distal conical shape, mimicking the effect of a minimally inflated balloon. They are positioned with this portion partially outside to the mouth of the AC to minimize the step-up between the inner diameter of the AC and the outer diameter of the MC (ledge reducing effect). The WEDGE™ Microcatheter (Terumo-Neuro, U.S./Japan) is FDA approved and available in Europe with a length of 160 cm that allows easier distal navigation of the SOFIA™ 6F (length = 131 cm, inner lumen 0.070″) but can also be used in combination with other, similarly sized catheters, such as the RED72 (inner lumen 0.072″). It is a 0.021 MC, 160 cm long with a tip length of 1.5 cm and is positioned inside the AC using 3 radiopaque tip markers (Fig. 7.10). Because of lacking distal reinforcement, the WEDGE is not recommended for deployment of SRs. Penumbra has launched a similar support device, the SENDit™ technology system, specifically designed for the use with RED72 catheters that comes preloaded with 0.014″ wire to reduce the ledge for easier distal tracking of the AC (Fig. 7.11).

A conically shaped MC tip can also be of great value when attempting to pass a highly stenotic (filiform) or even occluded ICA with a large AC as it minimizes vessel wall trauma and the possibility of creating a dissection.

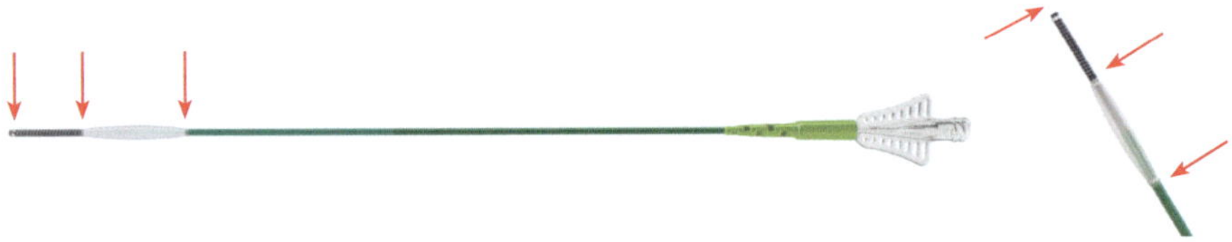

Fig. 7.10 WEDGE (Image courtesy MicroVention, Terumo). This microcatheter has a conical (distal and proximal) end, creating a fusiform shape and was primarily developed as an access tool for the SofiaPlus catheter to overcome obstacles such as the take-off of the ophthalmic artery from the clinoid ICA where often large-bore ACs get stuck and can cause damage. This MC is placed inside the Sofia, flushed (as is the Sofia) and advanced over a 0.014″ GW (Traxcess, Synchro). It has three tip markers (arrows) and must be positioned properly in order to reduce the ledge between inner lumen of the Sofia and outer diameter of the MC (achieved only when the proximal 2 makers are aligned with the Sofia tip in between). While the MC is long enough and also has a good trackability into the M2 territory, its use for stent retriever deployment is discouraged by the manufacturer. Its distal tip is not reinforced and stent retriever withdrawal may cause damage and complications. This required exchange for another 0.021 MC to switch to stent retriever in cases where aspiration fails is a disadvantage

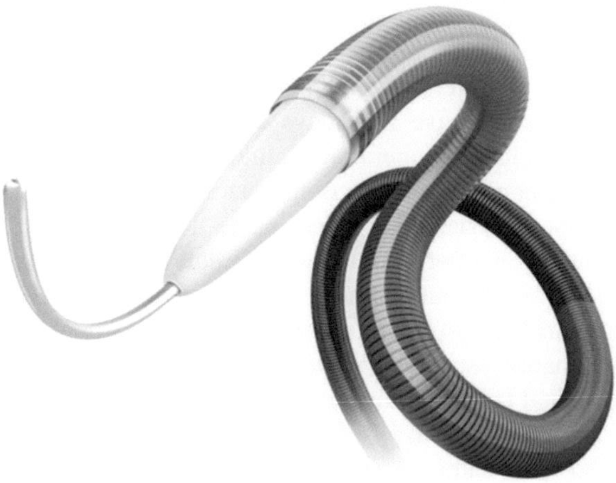

Fig. 7.11 The SENDit technology (Image courtesy Penumbra). Newly introduced by Penumbra, is compatible with a 0.014″ GW, has a tapered tip that occupies 99% of the lumen of a RED72 AC, and thus facilitates advancement and navigation in tortuous anatomy by eliminating the ledge between MC and AC typically responsible for getting stuck in the carotid syphon, e.g., at the ophthalmic artery take off

Following the concept of "ledge reduction" in coaxial systems, Route 92 Medical (San Mateo, CA) developed the conically tapered T7 Tenzing™ [186] that allows advancing the AC to the target site without using a GW [187].

Different from the initial concept that the tip of the aspiration catheter should aim to match the size of the M1 (average 2.6 mm) to maximize aspiration force and efficiency, a more recent alternative suggestion is to slightly undersize the catheter instead, and thus to create some space around of the catheter tip for a better aspiration effect. Apart from the original pump provided by Penumbra (Penumbra Max) and an improved version (Penumbra Jet Engine, Fig. 7.8), Stryker (Medela, AXS), Medtronic (Riptide), and Imperative Care (Zoom POD and PUMP) also provide aspiration pumps [188]. Alternatively, as mentioned above, manual aspiration using so-called vacuum-lock syringes can be applied as well, is easy to perform, and can be equally efficient in clots that develop intraprocedural during or after stenting. This technique should be considered, especially in a clinical setting where TE is not provided as a routine 24/7 service. Interestingly, a recent study demonstrated superior efficiency of this technique versus ADAPT when combined with SRs versus ADAPT [156].

For some time, the debate which TE technique, stent retriever or direct aspiration, is more efficient has resulted in a number of comparison trials without clearly demonstrating superiority of one technique versus the other [141, 148, 189–193]. Operators should use what they feel most comfortable with, and also be flexible if one method fails. Both techniques are associated with the risk of causing dissection, spasm and endothelial injury. Animal studies have shown that both aspiration and the use of SRs can cause damage to the arterial wall [194]. It should be noted though that nowadays stent retrievers are almost always used in some sort of combination with aspiration either via the side arm of a Y-connector (RHV) of the main guide or the intermediate (aspiration) catheter. The so-called *Solumbra-Technique* (Solitaire plus Penumbra) and several modifications of it termed "hybrid thrombectomy" are widely applied today [126, 195, 196].

In this context, it is interesting to note that the latest trend in the industry is to offer both TE options, e.g., Penumbra, the company pioneering clot aspiration technology, offers meanwhile a retrieval device while vendors originally focusing on SRs only have nowadays also aspiration kits in their portfolio (Medtronic, Stryker). Ideally, operators should be familiar with both techniques and use them not in a competitive but complementary manner.

Clot material that forms inside a carotid stent, either during deployment or immediately after, should be preferably aspirated, e.g., using a 5F or 6F Sofia catheter to avoid entanglement between stent and SR with possible dislocation [82]. Similarly, for M1 occlusions and in cases where aspiration fails, it may be more reasonable, especially when repeated attempts become necessary, to place a large AC distal to the carotid stent and use a stent retriever instead.

While the industry continues to develop larger access tools such as so-called super-bore catheters, the catheter's tip also has been a target of modifications. So has Imperative Care adopted the beveled tip configuration ("angled tip") from interventional cardiology and introduced a family of four Zoom™ catheters (Imperative Care, Fremont, CA) in various sizes (from "35 to 71") as well as their own pump system [197]. The company also offers a super-bore access catheter 0.088″, and early clinical results are promising (Fig. 7.12).

A recent development in the aspiration technology is the introduction of oscillating aspiration force to fragmentate the clot material and facilitate its aspiration.

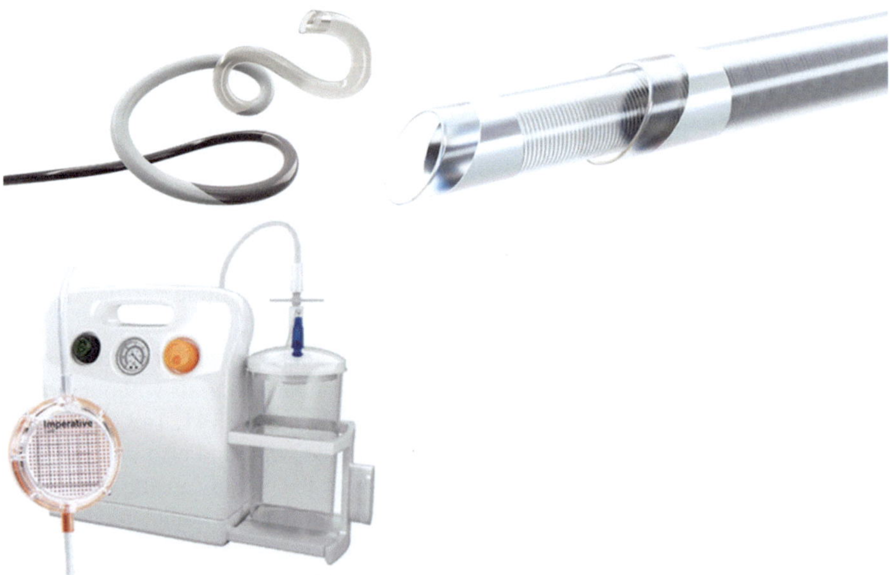

Fig. 7.12 Zoom aspiration catheters (Image courtesy Imperative care). While aspiration catheters with beveled tips are known in interventional cardiology, they have been new to the neuroendovascular field. The new Zoom family of ACs offers a range from the Zoom™ 88 (0.088, "Super-bore") angled tip (beveled) main guiding catheter and four aspiration catheters (71, 55, 45 and 35) all with a beveled tip. The company also offers its own pump, Zoom™ POD (left)

This avenue is pursued by several companies, including Penumbra and a start-up (RapidPulse™ Cyclic Aspiration System, CA) [198]. A different possible alternative is the future use of ultrasonic maceration of clot material into minute, non-occlusive particles, a technique called *Sonothrombolysis* [199]. However, due to conflicting results in terms of efficacy (CLOTBURST study), the method is currently not recommended by the American Heart Association while modified versions of the technique are currently tested in animal experiments [199–201].

7.3.3 Balloon Guiding Catheters (BGCs)

The use of balloon guiding catheters (BCGs) in patients undergoing TE allows for temporary blockage of blood flow during the procedure and has been suggested by many but is not regularly practiced by all operators [149, 202–211]. This controversy is mainly based on the added technical difficulties to place a usually stiffer guiding catheter into the CCA, especially in diseased arteries with tortuous and difficult access anatomy. The Cello™ (Medtronic), one of the initial BGCs, available in 8 and 9F has been advocated as initial access tool for TE for some time. However, it provides limited trackability and stability so that its placement could easily prolong the procedure time [210], or make access sometimes even impossible (author's experience). Newer BCGs, such as the 8F Flowgate-2™ (Stryker Neurovascular, Fremont, CA) or the Bobby™ (Terumo-Neuro, U.S./Japan) [208] (Figs. 7.13 and 7.14) provide better navigability and support while accepting larger intermediate catheters (Flowgate2 inner lumen = 0.084″, Bobby = 0.086″ vs. 8F Cello = 0.075″) which will likely contribute to a wider use of BGCs [146].

In general, some operators continue to perform TEs without BGC while others use them only under certain circumstances such as tandem occlusions (ICA plus M1).

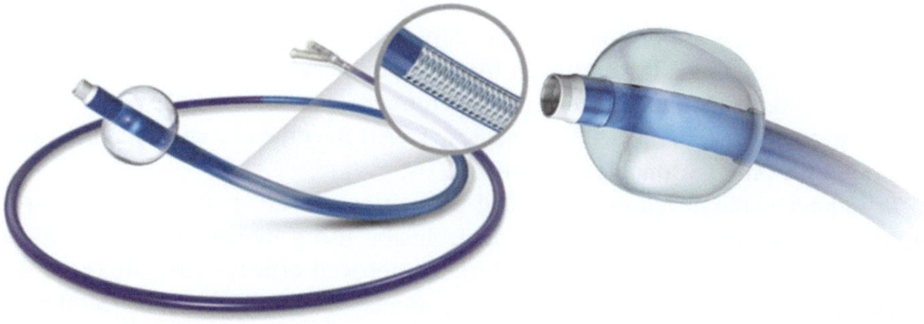

Fig. 7.13 Flowgate2 balloon guiding catheter (BGC, Image courtesy Stryker). The Flowgate 2 is an 8F, second-generation BGC with an improved design and better trackability that comes in 85 and 95 cm length. It could be used for TE in general or tandem occlusions (ICA plus M1) and has inner a lumen of 0.084″ which allows to deliver certain aspiration catheters distally, e.g., CAT6 or CAT5 (Stryker) for either direct contact aspiration or deployment of a stent retriever. The CAT system from Stryker also has a particularly tapered microcatheter (AXS Offset) which facilitates navigating a CAT5 into a distal position in tortuous anatomy

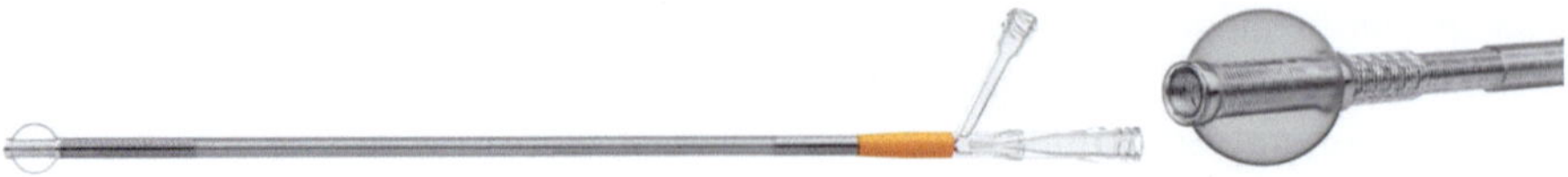

Fig. 7.14 Bobby balloon guiding catheter (Image courtesy TerumoNeuro): This recently introduced balloon guided catheter is more flexible and has a better trackability than the older generations of BGC. It comes in 95 cm and has an inner lumen of 0.086″ and accepts large-bore ACs like the Sofia 6F (not compatible with Flowgate2) and others which will likely contribute to a wider use of BGC for CAS in general but specifically for the treatment of acute tandem occlusions

Because of the advent of aspiration techniques, the risk of clot fragment embolism into the distal circulation has decreased which likely contributed to the reluctance of some operators to technically complicate an otherwise often straight forward procedure. In the author's personal practice, BGCs were rarely used for TEs, including tandem occlusions. Interestingly, new research has shown that placement of both, a large-bore AC and a BGC may adversely affect the outcome after TE due to possible blockage of collateral flow, increased penumbra and reduced back pressure [212]. More data is needed to clarify the pros and cons of using routinely BGCs, in particular in combination with large-bore aspiration catheters.

In elective ICA stenting where the use of either distal protection devices (filters) or proximal flow reversal using the MoMa™ system (Medtronic) is part of the procedure (standard of care), the use of a BGC may also be considered a valuable alternative.

A similarly modified concept is the recently introduced Walrus™ (Q'Apel Medical, Fremont, CA) catheter, available in 8F with a 0.087″ inner diameter, a 11 mm distal balloon and a 12 cm distal portion with variable stiffness [203, 213]. This catheter is available in the US and has been recently launched in Europe. Capuzzo et al. [213] described its use for achieving flow reversal by simple backflow from an opened three-way stopcock with 100% technical success and no ischemic complications in 105 patients. While flow reversal techniques using transfemoral access are promising, especially with modern BGC, the fundamental problem of navigating a large catheter through a diseased arch and CCA in patients with advanced plaque-laden atherosclerosis remains. In some of these patients who are not suitable CEA or TFCAS candidates, TCAR may then be considered a valuable if not the only reasonable alternative [214].

In summary, the development of 2nd-generation carotid stents, modern neuroprotection systems including proximal occlusion using modern BGCs and flow reversal combined with EPDs have further improved efficacy and safety of the procedure and widened the spectrum of patients. Elective CAS has become an important valuable alternative to open surgery. However, the general appeal of CAS is its minimal invasiveness and simplicity which should not necessarily be compromised by overloading its technical aspects with more add-on tools and devices. The dramatic recent evolution of mechanical thrombectomy (TE) in the treatment of AIS has resulted in a major shift in the management of the patients with LVOs caused by ICA stenosis or occlusion. Therefore, knowledge and skills in using various TE techniques become more relevant as contributing factors to the overall safety of patients undergoing CAS.

7.3.4 Pre- and Postprocedural Medication

Medical treatment of patients with cardiovascular diseases is an integral part of their clinical management and includes the treatment of hypertension, diabetes mellitus, lipid abnormalities as well as life style adjustments, such as smoking cessation and measures to reduce overweight. A detailed discussion of these aspects is, however, beyond the scope of this chapter.

Peri-procedural antiplatelet medication, on the other hand, plays a major role in the management of patients with carotid artery disease when undergoing CAS [215–217]. In absence of sufficient Level 1 evidence, the current recommendation of the Society of Vascular Surgery is the administration of 325 mg acetylsalicylic acid (ASA) and 75 mg clopidogrel (Plavix) daily at least 3 days prior and until 4 weeks after the procedure [215]. This combination of acetylsalicylic acid (ASA) and a $P2Y_{12}$ receptor inhibitor, known as dual antiplatelet therapy (DAPT) has become a mainstay for pre- and postprocedural platelet inhibition for elective CAS as well as for secondary stroke prevention [218]. In the neuroendovascular community, a premedication period with DAP drugs of at least 5 days is preferred [67]. In addition, testing the platelet inhibition using Verify Now or the Multiplate®-Test (Roche, Basel, Switzerland) is typically performed on the day before treatment in order to ensure safety of the procedure. In cases where the patient's response to DAP is insufficient, adjustments, e.g., dose increase of clopidogrel from 75 to 150 mg are usually recommended (lack of ASA response is possible but exceedingly rare). If retesting continues to show insufficient inhibition even with a higher dose, switch to alternative drugs such as prasugrel (Effient) with a loading dose of 60 mg, maintenance of 5–10 mg daily (depending on body weight) is suggested. Retesting post-procedure, although not performed by many operators, can be helpful as the response to clopidogrel often fluctuates and sufficient platelet inhibition pre-procedure does not always translate into the same during the post-procedure period (author's personal experience).

Clopidogrel, is a second-generation thienopyridine that selectively and irreversibly inhibits the P2Y12 ADP receptor and prevents platelet activation [219]. It is widely used in interventional cardiology and neuroradiology, and its response variability with "high on-treatment platelet reactivity" (HTPR) [220, 221], also called low or non-responder rate between 25% and 30% is a major drawback. It has been associated with an increased risk of cerebrovascular ischemic events [222–226] and triggered the search for more stable and stronger inhibitors of platelet activity.

Prasugrel (Effient), a third-generation thienopyridine is an irreversible P2Y12 ADP receptor antagonist, and like clopidogrel, a prodrug that requires activation in the liver in order to develop antiplatelet activity [227, 228]. On the other hand, it is rapidly absorbed and its active metabolites peak at 30 min. Even though clopidogrel and prasugrel are equipotent inhibitors on a molecular level [224], prasugrel produces higher concentrations of its active metabolites than does clopidogrel (15%). This and its more favorable pharmacokinetic profile produce a faster and stronger platelet inhibition [228]. In addition, it has less interindividual response variability compared to clopidogrel, and non-responders are extremely uncommon. While prasugrel has demonstrated clinical benefit over clopidogrel, it can also be associated with a higher bleeding risk [227] and should be given only with caution to patients over 75 years, with a known risk factors for intracranial hemorrhage and / or less than 60 kg body weight [229, 230] where a reduced dose (5 mg daily) is suggested.

Ticagrelor (Brilinta) is a metabolite that noncompetitively and reversibly inhibits P2Y12 receptors [230, 231]. The most important difference from other P2Y12 antagonists is that it is not a prodrug which needs to be metabolized for its inhibition effect. It has linear pharmacokinetics due to its high protein binding rate which reduces individual differences in efficacy and the antiplatelet activity begins rapidly after oral administration. In case of any bleeding or side effects, the efficacy disappears quickly after discontinuation of the drug [230]. In studies, the probability of high platelet activity during the procedure was reported to be between 1.5% and 4% in those receiving ticagrelor [8, 9]. This rate is quite low compared to clopidogrel.

Cangrelor (Kengreal), a nonthienopyridine adenosine triphosphate analogue, is another novel potent direct P2Y12 inhibitor which does not need conversion into an active metabolite, is immediately active after intravenous infusion, and has a half-life of 3–6 min. Its pharmacokinetics make it particularly well-suited for acute stent placement in the management of tandem occlusions for the treatment of acute stroke. A recent study comparing its use versus aspirin monotherapy and GP IIb/IIIa receptors in emergent CAS found lower odds of favorable clinical outcomes with cangrelor treatment compared to GPIIb/IIIa inhibitors [232].

Eptifibatide (Integrilin) is a cyclic peptide derivative that reversibly binds the GP IIb/IIIa receptors with subsequent inhibition of platelet aggregation and thrombus formation. It is FDA approved for coronary interventions [233] but has also been increasingly implemented in neuroendovascular practice for bridging to standard DAP in emergent carotid artery stenting during TE, e.g., in tandem occlusions. The intraprocedural administration of a IIb/IIIa inhibitor (GPIIb/IIIa), either in combination with 300–500 mg i.v. ASA or without has been historically the only available option in tandem occlusions [232, 234]. Heparin is usually avoided in these cases. This regimen has also been applied in the author's clinical practice.

The important role of DAPT for CAS has been addressed in a number of studies [67, 215, 221, 223, 225, 235]. While there is little doubt about the role of ASA, clopidogrel as the main P2Y12 inhibiting component has been increasingly replaced by newer generations of antiplatelet drugs (one indirect and two direct inhibitors). They are faster acting, stronger (prasugrel) and reversible (ticagrelor, cangrelor). The associated increased bleeding risk, however, must be balanced against their clinical benefits. One way to optimize monitoring of these patients would be testing the patient in the post-procedure period.

This is relevant not only for elective CAS but also for emergent scenarios where rapid inhibition can be crucial and time for dose adjustments and retesting is not available. Several recent publications report the use of ticagrelor or cangrelor for CAS, including in patients with tandem occlusions undergoing acute thrombectomy [216, 236–243]. The so-called Crash Loading (DAP < 1 day) does not necessarily cause more ischemic or hemorrhagic complications if patients are carefully selected and monitored [67].

While the need for pre- and periprocedural DAP is well established, little consensus exists which regimen for how long should be followed after CAS [217] which is in part due to the availability of several similar drugs with slightly varying pharmacokinetics and side effects as well as a significant heterogeneity in current practice [244]. An analysis of a large national US database showed that prolonged DAPT is associated with lower rate of readmissions for stroke but also a higher rate of hemorrhagic complications, specifically extracranial bleedings [217]. To better assess these risks versus benefits associated with a specific type and duration of antiplatelet medication, prospective data (RCTs) is needed.

In summary, periprocedural DAPT as a means to prevent ischemic complications post CAS is well established in the clinical management of carotid artery disease treated with carotid stents. While relatively clear recommendations for the premedication of patients undergoing CAS before CAS exist, such consensus for the postprocedural period, especially in terms of duration (4 weeks, 3 months?) has not been reached due to lacking Level 1 evidence. Thus, especially prospective data from RCT for elective and acute CAS is warranted.

7.3.5 Complications of CAS

While in 2025, CAS can generally be considered a relatively safe procedure if performed by experienced hands, precautions in terms of periprocedural medications and the use of intraprocedural EPDs must be taken. Nevertheless, as with any other medical procedure, complications do occur [245–252] and always will. When performing endovascular procedures in an arterial segment that is upstream to the most sensitive organ of the human body, the crucial aspect is that every measure was taken and/or considered to minimize the individual risk for a given patient. Factors that appear to have major influence on the complication rate during CAS are age, lesion length, and morphology as well as tortuosity index [245]. While patient's age (e.g., >80 years) has been traditionally considered the most important risk factor, some recent evidence suggests that unfavorable anatomy and anatomic variations including kinking, coiling, and severe tortuousities may play an even greater role [246, 252]. Therefore, careful studies of arterial anatomy prior to CAS for optimized patient selection are crucial in avoiding and minimizing adverse events and complications. In addition to intraprocedural complications, in some studies the majority of neurologic events occurred in the post-procedure period emphasizing the need for attentive observation immediately and at least during 14 days after stenting [247]. Interestingly, the degree of the stenosis (>90% vs. <90%) does not seem to have a significant influence on the complication rate [251]. With continuous advancements in imaging that allow better lesion characterization, and thus patients selection, optimized medical management and further improved embolic protection, future reduction of complications associated with CAS can be expected.

7.4 Illustrative Cases

7.4.1 Case 1: Elective ICA Stenting

A 72-year-old patient with intermittent left sided TIAs was referred from the department of vascular surgery for elective stenting due to the "high" location of his right ICA stenosis and was therefore considered not an ideal candidate for surgery. He was prepared with dual antiplatelet medication, 150 mg ASA and 75 mg clopidogrel daily and underwent testing (Multiplate Analyzer, Roche, Germany) the day before his procedure which showed a good response to both receptors (ASPI, ADP).

The patient's right femoral artery was accessed under general anesthesia, and an 8F short sheath was introduced. The patient received a 2000 IU bolus of heparin after which the activated clotting time (ACT) was monitored to maintain a level of 200–250 throughout the procedure. A 90 cm, 6–8F NeuronMax (NM, Penumbra) catheter was loaded with a 125 cm 5F MP (Multipurpose) Tempo (Cordis) catheter and a 0.035 Glidewire (Terumo) and flushed using pressured saline bags and air-free tubing with RHVs (Y-connectors) and three-way stopcocks. It was then introduced and navigated into the right common carotid artery. After reaching the distal CCA, DSA runs of the extra- and intracranial ICA were performed to show the exact location, length, and morphology of the ICA stenosis as well as the status of the cerebral circulation. Then, the MP catheter was removed while continuous flushing of the NM catheter was maintained. A 7 × 40 mm WallStent was prepared, and then gently advanced over a 0.014″ Traxcess wire into the distal ICA without interfering with the irregular part of the ICA stenosis. The GW was kept with its end in the distal ICA, proximal to the petrous portion. Following reaching the landing zone distal to the stenosis, the stent was deployed by unsheathing the device under fluoroscopy while maintaining a stable position of the delivery system. Following full deployment of the stent, the delivery system was removed and control runs were performed using contrast injection through the side arm of the three-way stopcock (Fig. 7.15). Patency and wall apposition of the stent were assessed, and the cerebral circulation was evaluated for distal occlusions. Following waiting 10 minutes and obtaining a negative repeat control DSA, the catheter system was removed, and a closure device (7F EXOSEAL, Cordis) was used to achieve hemostasis. The patient was extubated and monitored in the PACU for another 2 hours. He showed no new neurological symptoms or other complications and was transferred to the neurological ward. His platelet inhibition was controlled the next day and after an uneventful course over another 24 h, the patient was discharged with continuous DAP 75 mg clopidogrel and 150 mg ASA for the following three months. The three months FU CTA confirmed stent patency without signs of intimal hyperplasia or restenosis, and his medication was discontinued.

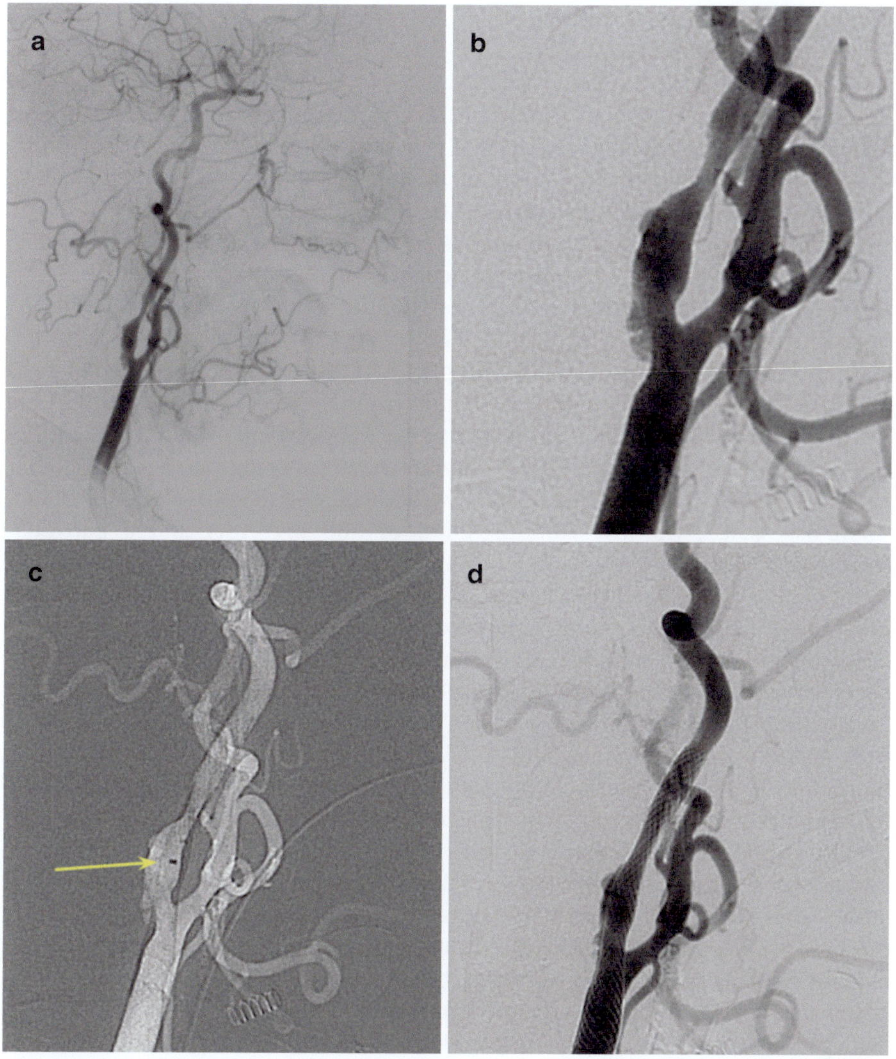

Fig. 7.15 (**a**–**d**): Symptomatic right ICA stenosis with elective carotid stenting. A 72 year-old male, heavy smoker with repeated TIAs and left-sided symptoms, CTA showed a "85% stenosis" of the right ICA. (**a**)**:** Right CCA injection, lateral view shows a severe (>70%) ICA stenosis. (**b**)**:** Magnified view reveals a highly irregular post-bifurcation segment. (**c**)**:** Road map shows of a 7 × 40 mm WallStent across the stenotic portion fully covering the diseased distal ICA with the proximal landing zone in the distal CCA. *Note in c:* the Sofia (arrow) inside the stent for "prophylactic aspiration" post-stenting. (**d**)**:** Final run shows good wall apposition and a fully patent stent until 10 minutes postprocedure

7.4.2 Cases 2 and 3: Emergent ICA Stenting in Tandem Occlusions

Below, two example cases of acute ischemic stroke caused by tandem occlusions are illustrated. Both patients were treated with the same basic approach as Case 1.

The second case showed a subtotal ICA occlusion caused by a concentric, filiform stenosis that caused stagnant flow in the distal cervical ICA (Fig. 7.16). The lesion was passed with a combination of the WEDGE and RED72 which allowed navigation into the distal cervical ICA while the main guide (Infinity) was kept in the CCA. Control injections confirmed the second occlusion by fresh clot in the clinoid ICA portion. The AC tip was navigated into the proximal portion of the clot using Road Map and ADAPT was performed using the Penumbra tubing and pump system. Control runs showed a recanalized ICA but a third thrombotic occlusion in the proximal M1-segment which, after further advancing the AC, was also successfully aspirated resulting into MCA recanalization (TICI 2c). The AC catheter was withdrawn, and the proximal ICA stenosis re-assessed. After i.v. administration of 500 mg ASA and a half-dose Integrilin bolus (90 mcg/kg), a 7 × 50 WallStent was deployed. Because of a significant residual stenosis, repeated (3×) post-dilatations using a 4.5 mm Maverick PTA catheter were performed. The procedure was then terminated, hemostasis achieved with EXOSEAL, and the patient was extubated. He was observed in PACU with blood pressure monitoring (systolic <140 mmHG) for 24 h before transfer to the stroke unit. The patient recovered well and showed a fully patent stent in a 3 months FU CTA.

The third case showed a complete occlusion of the ICA due to a heavily calcified plaque without any contrast flow into the cervical ICA (Fig. 7.17). This occlusion appeared irregular and rather firm suggesting a somewhat chronic nature and required multiple attempts to cross. Using a 0.014″ Traxcess, first with a straight, then a loop-shaped tip it was eventually possible to find a way through the heavily calcified firm material. After successful crossing, a PTA using a 1.5 mm and 3.5 mm Maverick balloon catheter (Boston Scientific) was performed first in order to create a channel wide enough for an AC to pass through. Because this was still not possible and re-occlusion appeared imminent, 500 mg ASA and an integrilin bolus (180 mcg/kg) were injected followed by deployment of a 9 × 30 mm WallStent. Then, a Sofia 6F loaded with a WEDGE MC was navigated into the right M1 segment where one direct aspiration was performed which resulted in MCA recanalization with TICI 2b. The AC was withdrawn, and a third PTA was performed followed by administration of 100 mcg nitroglycerin to improve the vasospasm. After the final run showed an acceptable 20–30% residual narrowing, the access site was closed with EXOSEAL, the patient extubated and transferred to the PACU for 24 h observation. CTA FU after 3 months documented stent patency.

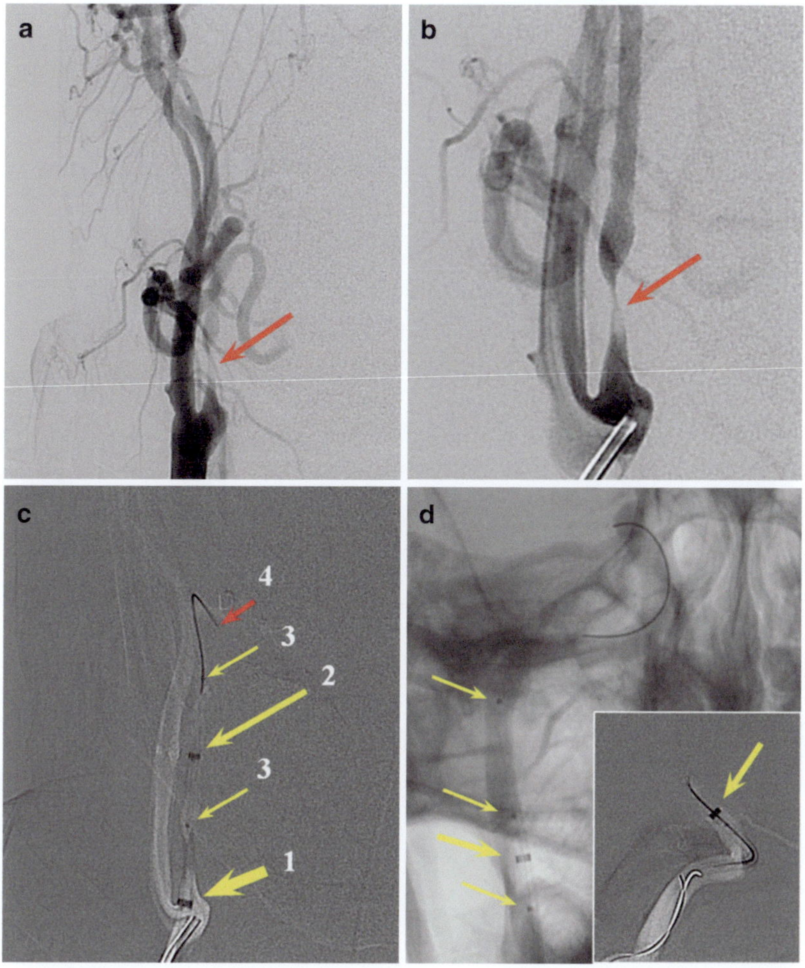

Fig. 7.16 (**a-h**): Case 2, subtotal ICA and M1 (tandem) occlusions with emergent ICA stenting. A 60-year old male with acute left-sided stroke. (**a**)**:** CCA injection shows a severe ICA stenosis (arrow) ICA severe stenosis and not much filling of the distal cervical ICA (subtotal occlusion). (**b**)**:** Proximal ICA injection reveals better the filiform but smooth stenosis with a normal distal lumen (arrow). (**c**)**:** The stenosis can be crossed with RED 72 (arrow) loaded with a WEDGE (short arrows) and a distal 0.014″ Traxcess wire (red arrow). (**d**)**:** RED72 navigated into the distal cervical ICA without difficulties. (*Note in* **c** and **d** *the triaxial catheter system*: NeuronMax: (1), RED72 (AC): (2), WEDGE: (3), Traxcess GW: (4). *Insert in* ***d:*** The tip of the AC is lodged into the first clot just distal the ophthalmic artery take-off from the ICA arrow. This is also the segment where large-bore ACs get often stuck due to the "ledge effect" when used with standard 0.021″ MCs.

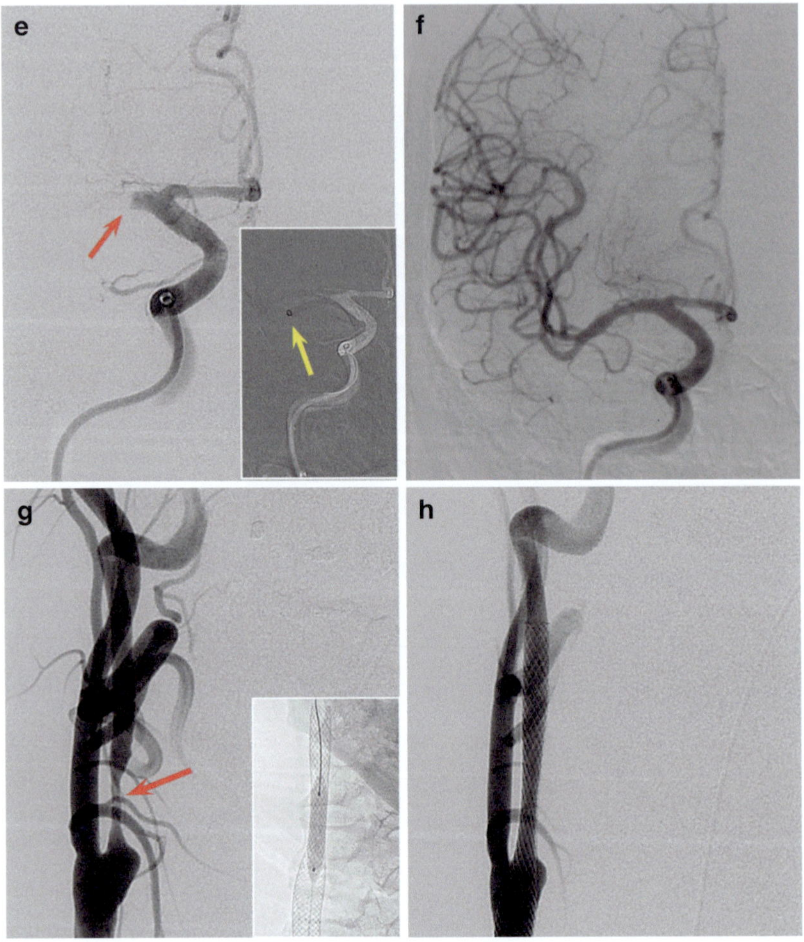

Fig. 7.16 (continued) (**e**)**:** ICA run post 1. aspiration in the cavernous portion shows now a 2nd, proximal M1 occlusion (arrow). The abrupt cut-off indicates fresh clot. *Insert:* the RED72 is navigated using same technique (coaxial over WEDGE) into the M1 segment (arrow, slipped further distal during aspiration). (**f**)**:** Control run through RED72 post 2. aspiration shows recanalized MCA. (**g**)**:** The proximal filiform stenosis appears meanwhile less severe due to "dottering" by the large-bore AC, however, is likely to re-occlude. Therefore, a 7 × 50 mm WallStent is deployed and post-dilated using a Maverick 4.5 mm balloon catheter (*Insert*). (**h**)**:** Final CCA run shows as a satisfactory result with close-to-normal luminal diameter and good distal run-off. CTA FU after 3 months confirmed stent patency

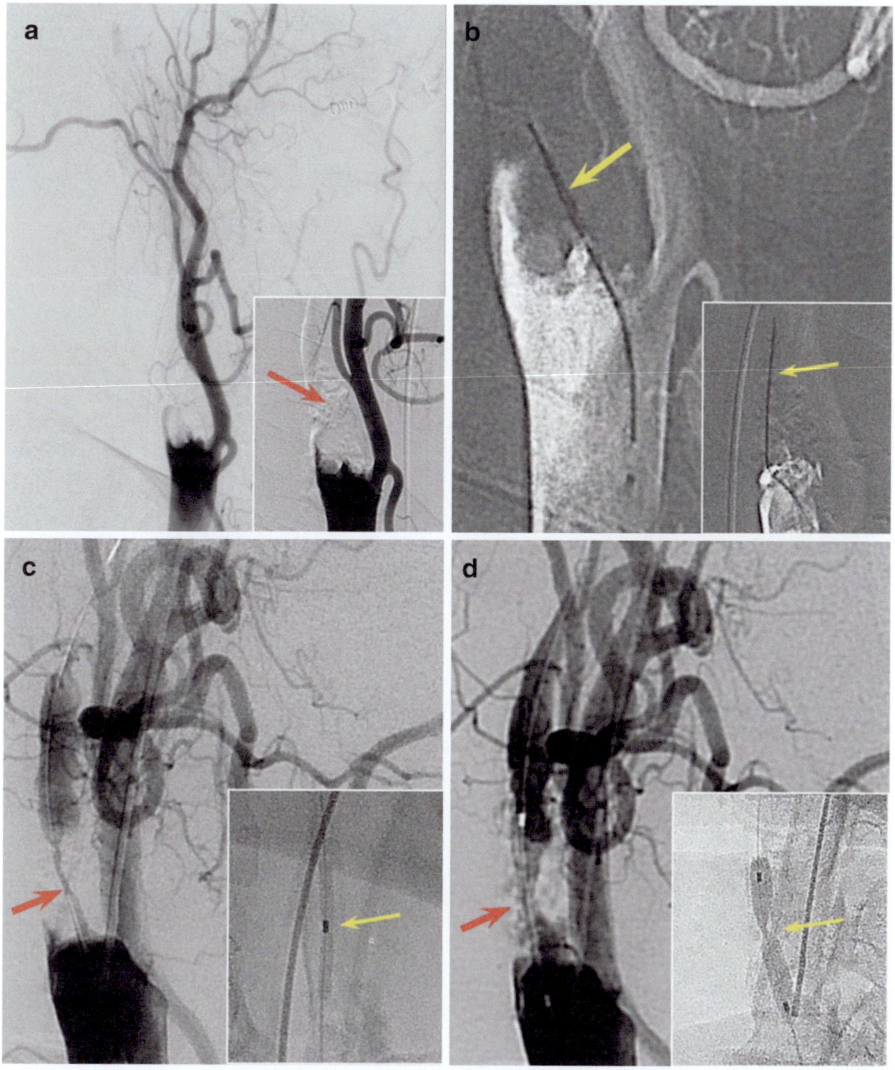

Fig. 7.17 (**a**–**j**): Case 3, complete ICA and M1 (tandem) occlusions with emergent ICA stenting. A 71-year-old male with acute left-sided stroke. (**a**)**:** Right CCA injections show complete ICA occlusion (ICA stump) with severely calcified plaque (Insert arrow). (**b**)**:** Road Map with 0.014″ Traxcess (arrow) shaped into a loop inside the plaque that is firm and difficult to pass through (Insert, arrow). (**c**)**:** Extremely narrowed, filiform channel (arrow) through the thick plaque after 1. PTA using 1.5 mm Maverick balloon (Insert, arrow). (**d**)**:** Slightly more enlarged, irregular lumen after 2. PTA with a 2.5mm Maverick (Insert, arrow).

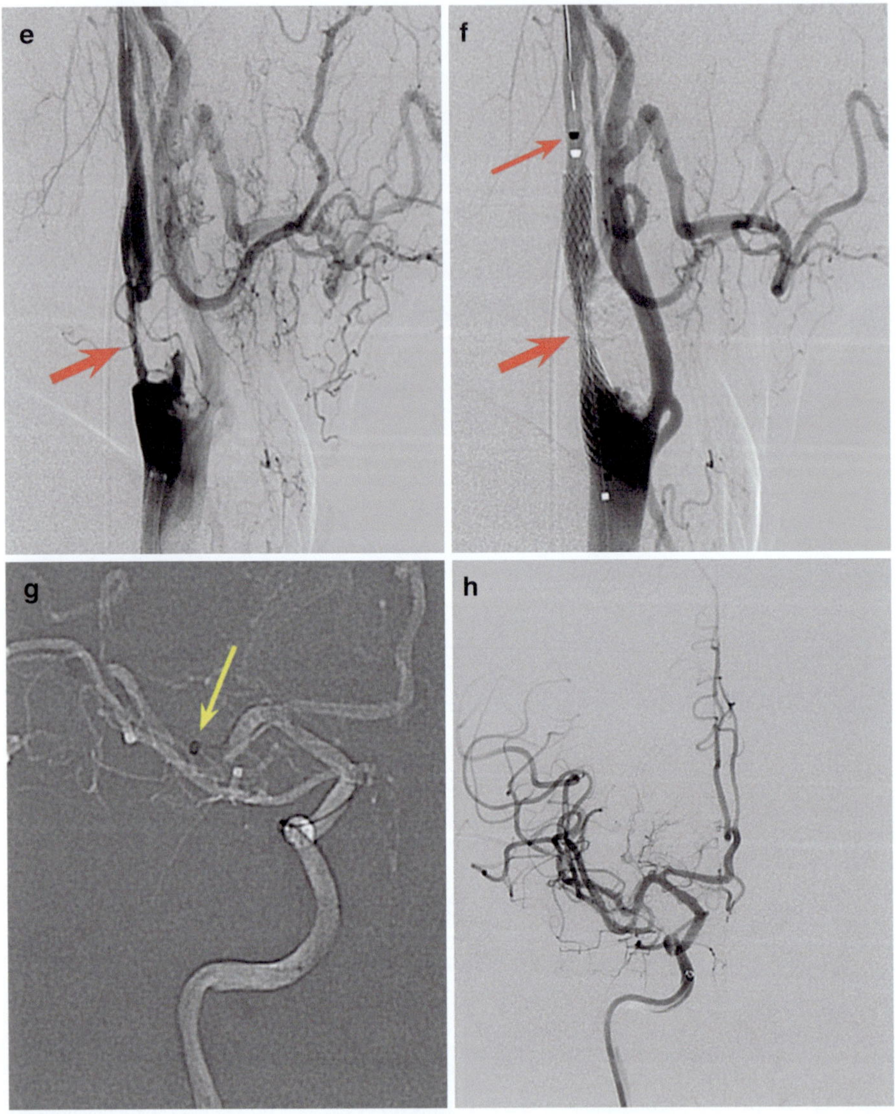

Fig. 7.17 (continued) (**e**)**:** Post 2. PTA run shows narrow channel in lateral view that would not allow to pass an AC. (**f**)**:** After deployment of a 9 × 30 mm WallStent through the stenosis (thick arrow), the Sofia (thick arrow), loaded with WEDGE, is navigated into the distal ICA. (**g**)**:** Road map shows the Sofia being positioned into the mid M1 segment (arrow) for aspiration. (**h–i**)**:** Post-aspiration control run shows recanalized MCA with TICI 2b.

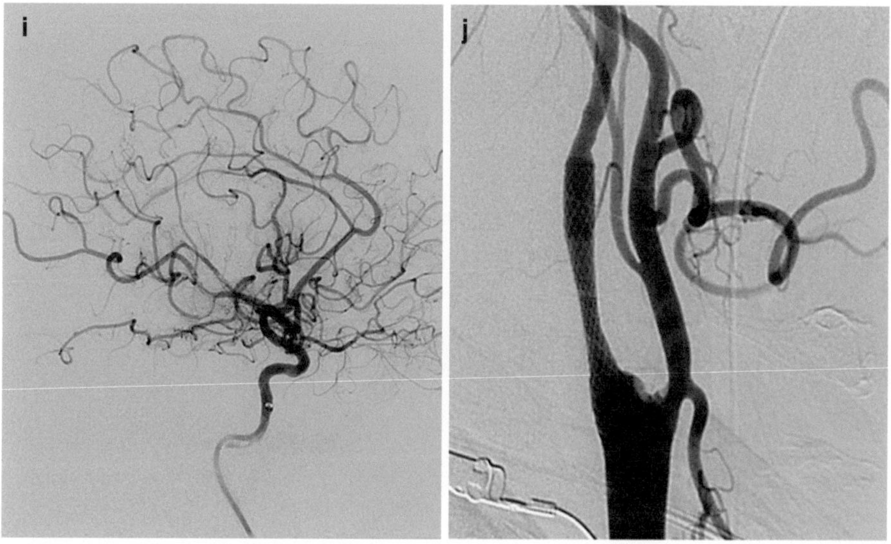

Fig. 7.17 (continued) (**j**): CCA injection after 3rd PTA of the proximal ICA stenosis with acceptable result (20–30% residual stenosis). Intermittent severe spasm post stenting and PTA was managed with i.a. injection of 100 mcg nitroglycerin. CTA FU after 3 months confirmed patency of the stent G. Benndorf

7.4.3 Case 4: Emergent ICA Stenting in CBS

A 53-year-old patient with a history of right hypopharyngeal cancer (planocellular carcinoma) and metastases to the right level II & III + left level II lymph nodes underwent treatment with chemotherapy and radiation. One year later, she was referred to the local ENT department with a recurrence and underwent a pharyngolaryngectomy. After one month, a CT scan showed that the patient had developed an abscess with perforation to the skin level and a fistula communicating with the oropharynx near the right carotid artery. Because she was now considered being at a significant risk for developing a carotid blow-out syndrome (CBS), the patient was consented for preventive carotid stenting. After she was loaded with DAP medication (ASA 300 mg and prasugrel 60 mg) the night before, transfemoral access using a 9F short sheath was obtained under GA. After a bolus of 1000 IU heparin, an 8F NeuronMax guiding catheter was then navigated into the right CCA using a 5F Tempo MP catheter over a 0.035″ Glidewire. A 2D-DSA showed an intact carotid lumen with a minimally decreased caliber and a small shallow outpouching at the distal CCA (level of bifurcation, Fig. 7.18). A 0.014″ guidewire was then advanced into the distal ICA under Road Map and a 6 × 50 mm Viabahn stent graft was introduced and deployed across the bifurcation. Control DSA showed full patency with good wall apposition of the stent. The previously documented small outpouching at the distal CCA was no longer visible. It also showed complete disappearance of

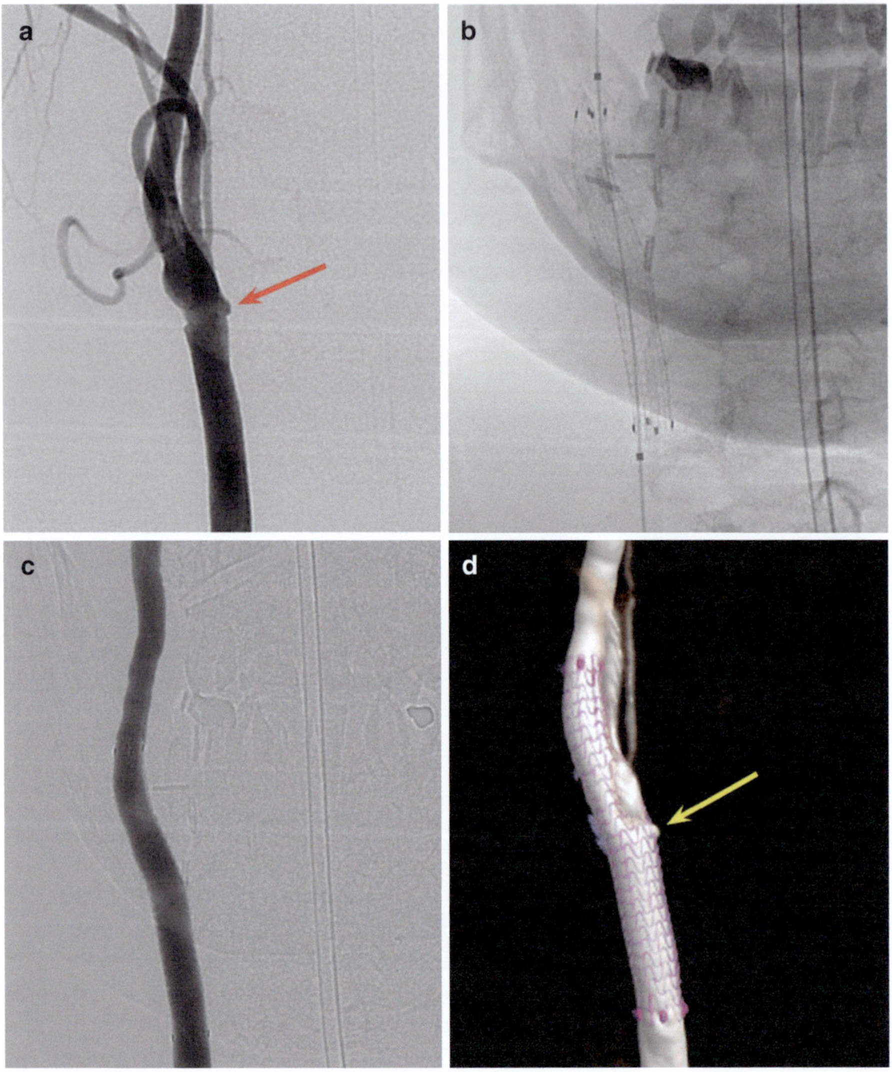

Fig. 7.18 (**a–d**): Case 4, risk of carotid blow-out syndrome (CBS) with emergent stenting. A 47-year-old female with a history of hypo-pharyngeal cancer (planocellular carcinoma) underwent chemo- and radiation therapy. Recurrence after one year with a new abscess and a fistula to skin level in close proximity to the carotid artery: Imminent risk of CBS. (**a**)**:** Right CCA injection shows a small shallow out-pouching (arrow) likely consistent with a pre-stage pseudoaneurysm. (**b**)**:** Post deployment of a 6 × 50 mm Viabahn, a non-subtracted view shows the fully opened stent graft. (**c**)**:** Control run post stenting shows patent ICA, no clot formations (until 22 min post deployment) and no longer filling of the small out-pouching. Note the missing ECA that is now blocked by the graft. This has usually no clinical consequences for the distal territory. (**d**)**:** 3D-DSA and fusion shows the stent graft covering the affected carotid portion with the small out-pouching

antegrade ECA flow which was compensated by collaterals. The intracranial circulation was assessed as normal, and the procedure was then terminated. After achieving hemostasis using an 7F EXOSEAL, the patient was extubated and woke up without sequelae. She did not experience bleeding episodes post stenting or side effects of the treatment. The patient was kept on DAP (150 mg ASA, 10 mg prasugrel) for the following 3 months and then kept on 80 mg of ASA indefinitely.

7.5 Comments and Practical Points

As detailed above, various stents for CAS are currently available among which DLSs will likely play an increasing role in the future as "protective stents" even though they "protect" not before implantation. As shown in 7.4, the use of EPDs and BGCs is, although generally recommended, not regularly practiced by all operators (including the author).

Further, no current consensus exists regarding the use of general anesthesia (GA). Even though, CAS can be performed as an outpatient procedure, even using TRA, many neurovascular centers with an established, well-functioning neuroanesthesia service may utilize GA for CAS, in particular in patients with acute ischemic stroke and LVOs. This is also the author's personal experience.

If a tandem occlusion is caused by an acute dissection that cannot be sufficiently reopened and repaired, prior or after TE, intentional permanent ICA occlusion to prevent further embolism can be a valid treatment option.

Technical and procedural details of the clot removal itself vary significantly between operators, including whether to use SR or AC first, and are left to the discretion and preference of the interventionist. Because direct aspiration is a relatively simple and fast method, the author prefers aspiration as first choice but also uses SR regularly whenever aspiration fails or recanalization remains incomplete.

During advancement of ACs loaded with a WEDGE, one must assure to keep correct positioning of the 2 catheters as the MC may slip back and for and lose its point of "maximum luminal occupation" inside the AC. In cases of difficult distal access for the AC, a "SR-anchoring technique" can also be used.

The duration of the applied vacuum during ADAPT may vary from the initial manufacturer's recommendation of 60–90 s to 3–5 min (author's preference). In order to fully engage a clot in the M1 and "cork" it into the mouth of the AC, longer aspiration can be useful.

Prompt return of blood flow (free flow) through the aspiration tubing is a sign of either the AC tip not being fully engaged with the clot or, the vacuum has already successfully removed it. The catheter should then be withdrawn and depending on the control, be re-advanced to the occlusion site. If the tip of the AC moves forward during aspiration, it is usually a sign that clot material is aspirated into the distal end of the catheter. No return of blood during aspiration usually indicates that the clot is efficiently "corked in" and will unlikely dislodge from the catheter tip when removed.

Some caution is advised during control runs via a large-bore catheter as applied high manual injection pressure may cause dislodgement and migration of residual clot material further distal and cause re-occlusions even when a BGC is being used.

Care must also be taken not to loose any clot material in the proximal Y-connector (at the main guiding catheter) when removing the AC with the thrombus "hanging" from its tip. In doubtful cases, the RHV should be inspected and if necessary, cleaned before continuing the procedure. The use of heparin is generally discouraged during TE and emergent CAS to reduce the risk of post-procedure intracranial hemorrhage.

If a SR is used, e.g., after failed aspiration, the AC should be placed as close as possible to the SR (distal ICA or M1) and simultaneous aspiration while withdrawing the SR should be applied.

The order of steps in tandem occlusion is a matter of debate, some operators would stent first and then try to remove the intracranial clot, others and likely the majority, would first recanalize the anterior circulation and place the stent afterwards (if necessary). As shown in the second emergent case, this is not always possible and stenting first can be required to even allow distal access with ACs.

In cases with very hard clot or atherosclerotic material, stiffer guidewires may become necessary for successful crossing which can be done with 0.018″ or even 0.035″ wires. However, caution is advised as perforation may occur, complicating rapidly the clinical situation of the patient. Therefore, the author prefers 0.014 guidewires which are more flexible and easier to use with a "loop-tip" (J-eyed tip) which usually navigates better through irregular, calcified occlusions.

If emergent stenting is performed after TE, watchful-waiting for about 10–15 min before terminating the procedure and closing the puncture site is advisable in the author's experience, for two reasons. Firstly, in elderly patients with elevated intracranial bleeding risk, ASA either as monotherapy or combined with only a half-dose of integrilin (or other glycoprotein IIb/IIIa receptor inhibitors) may be sufficient to prevent clotting of the stent as described above. Performing 1–2 more control injections instead can be reasonable before giving the full dose of integrilin in case thrombus formation occurs. Secondly, an initial "clean" final run can be misleading and some patients may develop thrombus formation inside the stent with delay. In these patients, it may be advantageous to maintain femoral access and GA a little longer in order to act swiftly and perform rescue TE if necessary.

If in-stent clotting continues despite full dose medication, additional aspiration attempts may be quite effective in "vacuum-cleaning" the device.

Carotid blow-out syndromes (CBSs) are rare but potentially disastrous complications in patients undergoing surgery and radiation for H&N cancer. In cases with signs of imminent carotid perforation, prophylactive stenting, carefully balanced against its associated risks of thrombosis and ischemic complications, may be well justified to protect a patient from a difficult to control and potentially life-threatening bleeding (see above).

7.6 Transcarotid Access and Treatment of Carotid Stenosis (TCAR)

Transcarotid Artery Revascularization (TCAR), a novel alternative to both transfemoral CAS (TFCAS) procedures and CEA, has evolved within the last decade and has been increasingly practiced in the US [78, 214, 253–273]. TCAR is a hybrid procedure consisting of open surgical exposure of the carotid artery and endovascular stent placement. It is specifically performed in patients with an increased procedural risk of stroke and can be an effective choice for high-risk patients who may not be suitable candidates for traditional carotid endarterectomy or stenting.

The technique is in principle a stenting procedure that provides neuroprotection by proximal flow control and flow reversal [266]. It involves percutaneous access to the carotid artery through a small incision made at the base of the neck followed by temporary reversal of blood flow in the carotid artery prior to placing the ENROUTE®Stent (Silk Road Medical®, Sunnyvale, CA).

One of the unique aspects of TCAR is its key focus on neuroprotection during the procedure. The blood flow is temporarily reversed to protect the brain from plaque material and debris before the lesion is crossed with a wire or a device. After clamping proximally the CCA, the blood flow is reversed into the systemic circulation through an extracorporeal circuit by connecting the internal carotid artery (ICA) to the femoral vein. This significantly reduces the risk of stroke which is particularly relevant in high-risk patients with severe comorbidities, advanced age, or previous surgeries [214, 256, 260, 271]. The procedure can be performed with smaller incisions than CEA and typically results in less postoperative discomfort, a shorter recovery time, and a reduced risk of CN injuries when compared to traditional surgery. Therefore, TCAR may lead to faster recovery, reduced hospital stays, and the possibility of outpatient procedures. Patients often experience fewer complications like infection and scarring compared to open surgical methods. So far, TCAR has mostly been compared to transfemoral CAS in registries and showed in 3286 consecutive patients a lower in-hospital stroke (2.1% vs 4.2%), stroke (2.0 vs 3.1%), and death (0.5% vs 1.5%) [78].

In their meta-analysis comparing TCAR with CAS and CEA, Naazie et al. [274] found that TCAR was associated with a lower risk of stroke and death than TFCAS (1.33% vs 2.55%) suggested by two non-randomized studies. Four non-randomized studies showed a lower risk for CN injury but similar risks for stroke and death when compared with CEA. Two other recent meta-analyses mirror these results in terms of 30-day mortality and stroke risks but also emphasize the need for RCT and Level-1 evidence data [272–275]. Silk Road Medical has recently (in 2022) withdrawn TCAR from the European market but was acquired by Boston Scientific in 2024. According to the manufacturer, TCAR should only be performed under specific conditions, including minimal clavicle-carotid bifurcation distance of 5 cm, CCA diameter >6 mm, ICA diameter >4 mm and minimal CCA plaques. Other relative contraindications are severe carotid tortuousities, calcifications, or fresh thrombus. The most frequent technical complication has been sheath-placement related dissection in atherosclerotic vessels. When compared to transfemoral CAS, higher costs are currently another drawback of the technique [248].

It should be noted that TCAR may not necessarily be seen as a competitive but rather complementary treatment choice to CEA and TFCAS. Each procedure has specific indications and contraindications and as concluded from a Delphi Consensus, TCAR cannot replace CEA and TFCAS but should be considered for symptomatic patients >80 years and the treatment of restenosis following CEA/TFCAS [263].

References

1. Roffi M, Mathias K. History of carotid artery stenting. J Cardiovasc Surg. 2013;54(1):1–10.
2. Theron J. My history of carotid angioplasty and stenting. J Invasive Cardiol. 2008;20(4):E102–8.
3. Theron J, Guimaraens L, Coskun O, Sola T, Martin JB, Rufenacht DA. Complications of carotid angioplasty and stenting. Neurosurg Focus. 1998;5(6):e4.
4. Theron J, Courtheoux P, Alachkar F, Bouvard G, Maiza D. New triple coaxial catheter system for carotid angioplasty with cerebral protection. Am J Neuroradiol. 1990;11(5):869–74.
5. Mathias K. Perkutane Transluminal Katheterbehandlung supraaortaler Arterienobstruktionen. Angiology. 1981;3:47–50.
6. Vitek JJ, Raymon BC, Oh SJ. Innominate artery angioplasty. AJNR Am J Neuroradiol. 1984;5(1):113–4.
7. Kerber CW, Cromwell LD, Loehden OL. Catheter dilatation of proximal carotid stenosis during distal bifurcation endarterectomy. AJNR Am J Neuroradiol. 1980;1(4):348–9.
8. White CJ, Brott TG, Gray WA, Heck D, Jovin T, Lyden SP, et al. Carotid artery stenting: JACC state-of-the-art review. J Am Coll Cardiol. 2022;80(2):155–70.
9. Tanaka N, Martin JB, Tokunaga K, Abe T, Uchiyama Y, Hayabuchi N, et al. Conformity of carotid stents with vascular anatomy: evaluation in carotid models. AJNR Am J Neuroradiol. 2004;25(4):604–7.
10. Lal BK, Roubin GS, Rosenfield K, Heck D, Jones M, Jankowitz B, et al. Quality assurance for carotid stenting in the CREST-2 Registry. J Am Coll Cardiol. 2019;74(25):3071–9.
11. Castriota F, de Campos Martins EC, Liso A, Biamino G, Cremonesi A. Technical evolution of carotid stents. Interv Cardiol (London). 2008;3(1):74.
12. Stoeckel D, Pelton A, Duerig T. Self-expanding nitinol stents: material and design considerations. Eur Radiol. 2004;14(2):292–301.
13. Li L, Pan S, Zhou X, Meng X, Han X, Ren Y, et al. Reduction of in-stent restenosis risk on nickel-free stainless steel by regulating cell apoptosis and cell cycle. PLoS One. 2013;8(4):e62193–e.
14. Sheth S, Litvack F, Dev V, Fishbein MC, Forrester JS, Eigler N. Subacute thrombosis and vascular injury resulting from slotted-tube nitinol and stainless steel stents in a rabbit carotid artery model. Circulation (New York, NY). 1996;94(7):1733–40.
15. Vajda Z, Miloslavski E, Güthe T, Schmid E, Schul C, Albes G, et al. Treatment of intracranial atherosclerotic arterial stenoses with a balloon-expandable cobalt chromium stent (Coroflex Blue): procedural safety, efficacy, and midterm patency. Neuroradiology. 2010;52(7):645–51.
16. Patel NJ, Heuser RR. Which embolic protection device is ideal during carotid artery stenting? Catheter Cardiovasc Interv. 2018;92(6):1136–7.
17. Zidan M, Gronemann C, Lehnen NC, Bode F, Weller J, Petzold G, et al. Stenting with dual-layer CGuard stent in acute sub-occlusive carotid artery stenosis and in tandem occlusions: a monocentric study. Neuroradiology. 2024;66(9):1635–44.

18. Zidan M, Voss YL, Wolf M, Keil F, Brockmann C, Gronemann C, et al. The dual-layer CGuard stent is safe and effective in emergent carotid artery stenting and in tandem occlusions: a multi-centric study. Clin Neuroradiol. 2024; https://doi.org/10.1007/s00062-024-01455-7.
19. Bartolini B, Puccinelli F, Mosimann PJ, Hajdu SD, Veunac L, Michel P, et al. Evaluating the effectiveness and safety of the carotid Casper-RX stent for tandem lesions in acute ischemic stroke. J Neurointerv Surg. 2019;11(8):772–4.
20. Garriboli L, Pruner G, Miccoli T, Recchia A, Tamellini P, Jannello AM. Carotid artery stenting without embolic protection device: a single-center experience. J Endovasc Ther. 2019;26(1):121–7.
21. Setacci C, Speziale F, De Donato G, Sirignano P, Setacci F, Capoccia L, et al. Physician-initiated prospective Italian Registry of carotid stenting with the C-Guard mesh-stent: the IRON-Guard registry. Rationale and design. J Cardiovasc Surg (Torino). 2015;56(5):787–91.
22. Kedev S, Müller-Hülsbeck S, Langhoff R. Real-world study of a dual-layer micromesh stent in elective treatment of symptomatic and asymptomatic carotid artery stenosis (ROADSAVER). Cardiovasc Intervent Radiol. 2022;45(3):277–82.
23. Langhoff R, Schwindt A, Vajda Z, Gjoreski A, Faurie B, Kedev S, et al. Navigating complexity with low-crossing profile dual-layer micromesh carotid stent: implications for contemporary carotid artery stenting outcomes (ROADSAVER study insights). J Cardiovasc Surg. 2024;65(3):205–12.
24. Montorsi P, Caputi L, Galli S, Ravagnani PM, Teruzzi G, Annoni A, et al. Carotid Wallstent versus Roadsaver stent and distal versus proximal protection on cerebral microembolization during carotid artery stenting. JACC Cardiovasc Interv. 2020;13(4):403–14.
25. Silvestri O, Accarino G, Turchino D, Squizzato F, Piazza M, Bastianon M, et al. Mid-term results of an Italian multicentric experience with the roadsaver (TM) dual-layer carotid stent system. Healthcare (Basel). 2024;12(1):120.
26. Vanzin JR, de Castro-Afonso LH, Santos MN, Manzato LB, Nakiri GS, Monsignore LM, et al. Casper vs. closed-cell stent: carotid artery stenting randomized trial. Clin Neuroradiol. 2021;31(3):843–52.
27. Angiology—Carotid Artery; New Carotid Artery Study Findings Recently Were Reported by Researchers at University of Arizona (Which embolic protection device is ideal during carotid artery stenting?). Obesity, Fitness & Wellness Week. 2018:3449.
28. Diaz O, Lopez G, Roehm JOF, De la Rosa G, Orozco F, Almeida R. The Casper carotid artery stent: a unique all metal micromesh stent designed to prevent embolic release. J Neurointerv Surg. 2018;10(2):133–6.
29. Bosiers M, Deloose K, Torsello G, Scheinert D, Maene L, Peeters P, et al. The CLEAR-ROAD study: evaluation of a new dual layer micromesh stent system for the carotid artery. EuroIntervention. 2016;12(5):e671–6.
30. Kahlberg A, Bilman V, Ardita V, Mascia D, Bertoglio L, Rinaldi E, et al. Contemporary results of carotid artery stenting using Low-profile dual-metal layer nitinol micromesh stents in relation to single-layer carotid stents. J Endovasc Ther. 2021;28(5):726–36.
31. Segawa M, Inoue T, Tsunoda S, Kanamaru T, Okubo S. Carotid endarterectomy for acute carotid thrombosis after carotid artery stenting with CASPER Rx(R) stent: a case report. Surg Neurol Int. 2023;14:25.
32. Wada T, Takayama K, Myouchin K, Oshima K, Tanaka T, Kichikawa K. Intraprocedural plaque protrusion during carotid artery stenting with a CASPER stent: a case report. J Neuroendovasc Ther. 2023;17(1):32–6.
33. Runck F, Maurer CJ, Berlis A. Complication rates using CASPER dual-layer stents for carotid artery stenting in acute stroke : a 3-year single center experience. Clin Neuroradiol. 2021;31(1):173–9.
34. Bosiers M, de Donato G, Deloose K, Verbist J, Peeters P, Castriota F, et al. Does free cell area influence the outcome in carotid artery stenting? Eur J Vasc Endovasc Surg. 2007;33(2):135–41. discussion 42–3

35. Wodarg F, Turner EL, Dobson J, Ringleb PA, Mali WP, Fraedrich G, et al. Influence of stent design and use of protection devices on outcome of carotid artery stenting: a pooled analysis of individual patient data. J Neurointerv Surg. 2018;10(12):1149–54.
36. Tigkiropoulos K, Sidiropoulou K, Abatzis-Papadopoulos M, Lazaridis I, Saratzis N. 12-Month outcomes of carotid artery stenting with CGuard MicroNET-covered stent: a single-center study in 113 patients. Angiology. 2023; https://doi.org/10.1177/00033197231213679.
37. Casana R, Tolva V, Odero A Jr, Malloggi C, Paolucci A, Triulzi F, et al. Safety and efficacy of the new micromesh-covered stent CGuard in patients undergoing carotid artery stenting: early experience from a single centre. Eur J Vasc Endovasc Surg. 2017;54(6):681–7.
38. de Borst GJ. Commentary to 'Safety and efficacy of the new micromesh-covered stent CGuard in patients undergoing carotid artery stenting: early experience from a single centre'. Eur J Vasc Endovasc Surg. 2017;54(6):688.
39. Klail T, Kurmann C, Kaesmacher J, Mujanovic A, Piechowiak EI, Dobrocky T, et al. Safety and efficacy of carotid artery stenting with the CGuard double-layer stent in acute ischemic stroke. Clin Neuroradiol. 2023;33(1):237–44.
40. Tigkiropoulos K, Papoutsis I, Abatzis-Papadopoulos M, Kousidis P, Mpismpos D, Melas N, et al. Thirty-day results of the novel CGuard-covered stent in patients undergoing carotid artery stenting. J Endovasc Ther. 2021;28(4):542–8.
41. Tigkiropoulos K, Nikas S, Ampatzis-Papadopoulos M, Sidiropoulou K, Stavridis K, Karamanos D, et al. One-year outcomes of CGuard double mesh stent in carotid artery disease: a systematic review and meta-analysis. Medicina (Kaunas). 2024;60(2):286.
42. Montorsi P, Galli S, Ravagnani PM, Tresoldi S, Teruzzi G, Caputi L, et al. Carotid artery stenting with proximal embolic protection via a transradial or transbrachial approach: pushing the boundaries of the technique while maintaining safety and efficacy. J Endovasc Ther. 2016;23(4):549–60.
43. Schönholz C, Yamada R, Montgomery W, Brothers T, Guimaraes M. First-in-man implantation of a new hybrid carotid stent to prevent periprocedural neurological events during carotid artery stenting. J Endovasc Ther. 2014;21(4):601–4.
44. Gray WA, Levy E, Bacharach JM, Metzger DC, Randall B, Siddiqui A, et al. Evaluation of a novel mesh-covered stent for treatment of carotid stenosis in patients at high risk for endarterectomy: 1-year results of the SCAFFOLD trial. Catheter Cardiovasc Interv. 2020;96(1):121–7.
45. Golarz SR, Gable D. Use of a Viabahn stent for repair of a common carotid artery pseudoaneurysm and dissection. Ann Vasc Surg. 2010;24(4):550.e11–3.
46. Patil M, Hassman BN, Johnson D, Thompson JR, Dowdall J, Cook JR. Post neck radiation cancer carotid pseudoaneurysm blowouts with Viabahn stent placement. Ann Vasc Surg. 2024; https://doi.org/10.1016/j.avsg.2024.08.015.
47. Kreiser K, Gröber I, Zimmer C, Storck K. Stent grafts in patients with carotid blowout syndrome: outcome and antiplatelet therapy in preventive versus emergency cases. Head Neck. 2018;40(11):2521–7.
48. Seraj FQM, Najafi S, Raaisi AA, Mirbolouk MH, Ebrahimnia F, Shamsi HP, et al. Treatment of traumatic direct carotid-cavernous fistula with a BeGraft-covered stent. Neurointervention. 2024;19(2):111–7.
49. Kischkel S, Grabow N, Puschel A, Erdle B, Kabelitz M, Martin DP, et al. Biodegradable polymeric stents for vascular application in a porcine carotid artery model: English version. Gefasschirurgie. 2016;21(Suppl 1):30–6.
50. Shen Y, Tang C, Sun B, Wu Y, Yu X, Cui J, et al. Development of 3D printed biodegradable, entirely X-ray visible stents for rabbit carotid artery implantation. Adv Healthc Mater. 2024;13(15):e2304293.
51. Cayne NS, Faries PL, Trocciola SM, Saltzberg SS, Dayal RD, Clair D, et al. Carotid angioplasty and stent-induced bradycardia and hypotension: impact of prophylactic atropine administration and prior carotid endarterectomy. J Vasc Surg. 2005;41(6):956–61.
52. Sangiorgi G, Colombo A. Embolic protection devices. Heart. 2003;89(9):990–2.

53. Cremonesi A. The SPIDER Embolic Protection Device performance evaluation in the carotid artery during percutaneous transluminal angioplasty and or stenting. J Invasive Cardiol. 2005;17(9):463–7.
54. Khan N, Murphy TP, Dubel GJ. Carotid artery stenting using distal embolic protection device. Med Health R I. 2005;88(3):96.
55. Zahn R, Ischinger T, Mark B, Gass S, Zeymer U, Schmalz W, et al. Embolic protection devices for carotid artery stenting. J Am Coll Cardiol. 2005;45(11):1769–74.
56. de Castro-Afonso LH, Abud LG, Rolo JG, dos Santos AC, de Oliveira L, Barreira CM, et al. Letter by de Castro-Afonso et al regarding article, "Operator's experience is the most efficient embolic protection device for carotid artery stenting". Circ Cardiovasc Interv. 2014;7(1):130.
57. Bauer C, Franke J, Bertog SC, Woerner V, Ghasemzadeh-Asl S, Sievert H. FiberNet—a new embolic protection device for carotid artery stenting. Catheter Cardiovasc Interv. 2014;83(6):1014–20.
58. D'Souza SB, Slovut DP, Bower TC, Bacharach JM. Do the advantages of the FiberNet((R)) embolic protection device translate into technical success and comparable event rates in carotid artery stenting? Neuroradiol J. 2009;22(1):80–5.
59. Giri J, Parikh SA, Kennedy KF, Weinberg I, Donaldson C, Hawkins BM, et al. Proximal versus distal embolic protection for carotid artery stenting: a national cardiovascular data registry analysis. JACC Cardiovasc Interv. 2015;8(4):609–15.
60. Hong N, Park JM, Kim SB, Son YJ. Flow arrest during carotid artery stenting with a distal embolic protection device: a single-center experience and clinical implications. J Cerebrovasc Endovasc Neurosurg. 2024;26(2):163–73.
61. Knappich C, Bohmann B, Kirchhoff F, Lohe V, Naher S, Kallmayer M, et al. Use of an embolic protection device during carotid artery stenting is associated with lower periprocedural risk. J Neurointerv Surg. 2024; https://doi.org/10.1136/jnis-2024-021722.
62. Stabile E, Esposito G. Operator's experience is the most efficient embolic protection device for carotid artery stenting. Circ Cardiovasc Interv. 2013;6(5):496–7.
63. Sugiu K, Martin JB, Pache JC, Gulmaraens L, Theron J, Rufenacht DA. Distal flow protection during carotid stenting. A prospective study to quantify the embolic debris retrieved in the internal carotid artery territory. Interv Neuroradiol. 1999;5(Suppl 1):47–50.
64. Parodi JC, Schönholz C, Mariano Ferreira L, Mendaro E, Ohki T. "Seat belt and air bag" technique for cerebral protection during carotid stenting. J Endovasc Ther. 2002;9(1):20–4.
65. Moukarbel GV, Sobieszczyk PS. Embolic protection devices. In: Owens CD, Yeghiazarians Y, editors. Handbook of endovascular peripheral interventions. Boston: Springer; 2012. p. 101–18.
66. Yilmaz M, Yabalak A. Carotid artery stenting with or without distal filter-type embolic protection device: a single center experience. J Bionic Memory. 2021;1(2–3):41–9.
67. Hajiyev K, Henkes H, Hellstern V, Khanafer A, Wendl C, Bazner H, et al. Is crash loading acceptable in carotid artery stenting?: Results of antiplatelet crash loading vs. semi-crash vs. elective loading in a large study population. Clin Neuroradiol. 2023;33(2):415–25.
68. Khan M, Qureshi AI. Factors associated with increased rates of post-procedural stroke or death following carotid artery stent placement: a systematic review. J Vasc Interv Neurol. 2014;7(1):11–20.
69. Texakalidis P, Letsos A, Kokkinidis DG, Schizas D, Karaolanis G, Giannopoulos S, et al. Proximal embolic protection versus distal filter protection versus combined protection in carotid artery stenting: a systematic review and meta-analysis. Cardiovasc Revasc Med. 2018;19(5 Pt A):545–52.
70. Parodi J, Bates MC, Ohki T, Schönholz C. The history of proximal carotid protection and flow reversal to prevent stent angioplasty embolization. Semin Vasc Surg. 2018;31(1):9–14.
71. Clair DG, Hopkins LN, Mehta M, Kasirajan K, Schermerhorn M, Schönholz C, et al. Neuroprotection during carotid artery stenting using the GORE flow reversal system: 30-day outcomes in the EMPiRE clinical study. Catheter Cardiovasc Interv. 2011;77(3):420–9.

72. Coppi G, Moratto R, Silingardi R, Rubino P, Sarropago G, Salemme L, et al. PRIAMUS—proximal flow blockage cerebral protectIon during carotid stenting: results from a multicenter Italian registry. J Cardiovasc Surg. 2005;46(3):219–27.
73. Bersin RM, Stabile E, Ansel GM, Clair DG, Cremonesi A, Hopkins LN, et al. A meta-analysis of proximal occlusion device outcomes in carotid artery stenting. Catheter Cardiovasc Interv. 2012;80(7):1072–8.
74. Ansel GM, Hopkins LN, Jaff MR, Rubino P, Bacharach JM, Scheinert D, et al. Safety and effectiveness of the INVATEC MO.MA® proximal cerebral protection device during carotid artery stenting: results from the ARMOUR pivotal trial. Catheter Cardiovasc Interv. 2010;76(1):1–8.
75. Nikas D, Reith W, Schmidt A, Duda S, Mathias K, Cremonesi A, et al. Prospective, multicenter European study of the GORE flow reversal system for providing neuroprotection during carotid artery stenting. Catheter Cardiovasc Interv. 2012;80(7):1060–8.
76. Hendriks JM, Zindlei JD, Van Dijk LC, Van Sambeek MRHM. Cerebral protection during percutaneous carotid intervention: which device should be used ? Acta Chir Belg. 2004;104(3):300–3.
77. Werner M, Scheinert D, Borghesi R, Cremonesi A, Rosenschein U, Scheinert S, et al. First clinical experience with the GARDEX EPD: a novel embolic protection device for carotid artery stenting. EuroIntervention. 2013;8(9):1026–32.
78. Kleindorfer DO, Towfighi A, Chaturvedi S, Cockroft KM, Gutierrez J, Lombardi-Hill D, et al. 2021 Guideline for the prevention of stroke in patients with stroke and transient ischemic attack: a guideline from the American Heart Association/American Stroke Association. Stroke (1970). 2021;52(7):e364–467.
79. Giri J, Yeh RW, Kennedy KF, Hawkins BM, Weinberg I, Weinberg MD, et al. Unprotected carotid artery stenting in modern practice. Catheter Cardiovasc Interv. 2014;83(4):595–602.
80. Montorsi P, Caputi L, Loaldi A, Parati E, Andreini D, Veglia F, et al. Microembolization during carotid artery stenting in patients with high-risk, lipid-rich plaque: a randomized trial of proximal versus distal cerebral protection. J Am Coll Cardiol. 2011;58(16):1656–63.
81. Omran J, Mahmud E, White CJ, Aronow HD, Drachman DE, Gray W, et al. Proximal balloon occlusion versus distal filter protection in carotid artery stenting: a meta-analysis and review of the literature. Catheter Cardiovasc Interv. 2017;89(5):923–31.
82. Fujita J, Hirotsune N, Matsuda Y, Hamasaki O, Fukuda S, Okada Y, et al. Important notes for preventing entrapment of distal filter-based embolic protection device in carotid artery stenting. Neurol Med Chir (Tokyo). 2024;64:382.
83. Li T, Zha Y, Bo L, Wirthlin DJ, Zhang Q. Surgical management for retained distal embolic protection device and fractured guidewire after carotid artery stenting. J Surg Case Rep. 2016;2016(6):rjw105.
84. Maramattom BV. Carotid dissecting aneurysm after carotid stenting with an embolic protection device. Neurol India. 2023;71(4):835–6.
85. Chmiel J, Tekieli L, Mazurek A, Czyz L, Musialek P. Filter protection in contemporary carotid artery stenting: consider limited protection. Postepy Kardiol Interwencyjnej. 2024;20(2):213–6.
86. Kohara K, Ishikawa T, Kobayashi T, Kawamata T. Retinal artery occlusion during carotid artery stenting with distal embolic protection device. Neuroradiol J. 2018;31(5):504–8.
87. Kim HJ, Rho MH. Massive cerebral microemboli after protected carotid artery angioplasty and stenting using a distal filter embolic protection device for a vulnerable plaque with a lipid rich necrotic core and intraplaque hemorrhage: a case report. Taehan Yongsang Uihakhoe Chi. 2020;81(3):739–45.
88. Finol E, Siewiorek G, Scotti C, Wholey M, Wholey M. Wall apposition assessment and performance comparison of distal protection filters. J Endovasc Ther. 2008;15:177–85.
89. Maleux G, Demaerel P, Verbeken E, Daenens K, Heye S, Van Sonhoven F, et al. Cerebral ischemia after filter-protected carotid artery stenting is common and cannot be predicted by the presence of substantial amount of debris captured by the filter device. Am J Neuroradiol. 2006;27(9):1830–3.

90. Macdonald S, Evans DH, Griffiths PD, McKevitt FM, Venables GS, Cleveland TJ, et al. Filter-protected versus unprotected carotid artery stenting: a randomised trial. Cerebrovasc Dis (Basel, Switzerland). 2010;29(3):282–9.
91. Kim SJ, Roh HG, Jeon P, Kim KH, Lee KH, Byun HS, et al. Cerebral ischemia detected with diffusion-weighted MR imaging after protected carotid artery stenting: comparison of distal balloon and filter device. Korean J Radiol. 2007;8(4):276–85.
92. Gray WA, Mehta M, Alani F, Kasirajan K, Begg RJ, Bacharach JM, et al. Use of a novel embolic filter in carotid artery stenting: 30-day results from the EMBOLDEN clinical study. Catheter Cardiovasc Interv. 2018;92(6):1128–35.
93. Langhoff R, Petrov I, Kedev S, Milosevic Z, Schmidt A, Scheinert D, et al. PERFORMANCE 1 study: novel carotid stent system with integrated post-dilation balloon and embolic protection device. Catheter Cardiovasc Interv. 2022;100(6):1090–9.
94. Petkoska D, Zafirovska B, Vasilev I, Saylors E, Sachar R, Kedev S. Transradial carotid artery stenting using double layer micromesh stent and novel post-dilation balloon with integrated embolic protection. Cardiovasc Revasc Med. 2024;63:43–51.
95. Bijuklic K, Wandler A, Hazizi F, Schofer J. The PROFI study (prevention of cerebral embolization by proximal balloon occlusion compared to filter protection during carotid artery stenting): a prospective randomized trial. J Am Coll Cardiol. 2012;59(15):1383–9.
96. Tatlı E, Buturak A, Doğan E, Alkan M, Sayın M, Yılmaztepe M, et al. Comparison of anti-embolic protection with proximal balloon occlusion and filter devices during carotid artery stenting: clinical and procedural outcomes. J Am Coll Cardiol. 2013;62(18):C76–C.
97. Cano MNMDP, Kambara AMMDP, de Cano SJFMD, Pezzi Portela LAMDP, Paes ÂTP, Costa JRMD, et al. Randomized comparison of distal and proximal cerebral protection during carotid artery stenting. JACC Cardiovasc Interv. 2013;6(11):1203–9.
98. Omran J, Al-Dadah AS, White CJ. Rebuttal regarding: proximal occlusion versus distal filter for cerebral protection during carotid stenting: the positive results of MO.MA trials. Catheter Cardiovasc Interv. 2018;92(5):1013–4.
99. Naylor R, Rantner B, Ancetti S, de Borst GJ, De Carlo M, Halliday A, et al. Editor's choice—European Society for Vascular Surgery (ESVS) 2023 Clinical Practice Guidelines on the management of atherosclerotic carotid and vertebral artery disease. Eur J Vasc Endovasc Surg. 2023;65(1):7–111.
100. Montorsi P, Cortese B, Cernetti C, Lanzellotti D, Di Palma G, Marchese A, et al. Transradial approach for carotid artery stenting: a position paper from the Italian Society of Interventional Cardiology (SICI-GISE). Catheter Cardiovasc Interv. 2021;97(7):1440–51.
101. Arakawa K, Harada K, Kajihara M, Kiyosawa R, Baba D, Oshima T. Anatomical navigational difficulties in transradial right carotid artery stenting with 7-F Optimo balloon guide catheter. Interv Neuroradiol. 2024; https://doi.org/10.1177/15910199241276906.
102. Wahood W, Ghozy S, Al-Abdulghani A, Kallmes DF. Radial artery diameter: a comprehensive systematic review of anatomy. J Neurointerv Surg. 2022;14(12):1274–8.
103. Campbell BC, Mitchell PJ, Yan B, Parsons MW, Christensen S, Churilov L, et al. A multicenter, randomized, controlled study to investigate EXtending the time for Thrombolysis in Emergency Neurological Deficits with Intra-Arterial therapy (EXTEND-IA). Int J Stroke. 2014;9(1):126–32.
104. McDowell MM, Ducruet AF. Time is brain: a critical analysis of the EXTEND-IA and ESCAPE trials. World Neurosurg. 2015;83(6):949–51.
105. Saver JL, Goyal M, Bonafe A, Diener HC, Levy EI, Pereira VM, et al. Stent-retriever thrombectomy after intravenous t-PA vs. t-PA alone in stroke. N Engl J Med. 2015;372(24):2285–95.
106. Jovin TG, Chamorro A, Cobo E, de Miquel MA, Molina CA, Rovira A, et al. Thrombectomy within 8 hours after symptom onset in ischemic stroke. N Engl J Med. 2015;372(24):2296–306.
107. Berkhemer OA, Fransen PS, Beumer D, van den Berg LA, Lingsma HF, Yoo AJ, et al. A randomized trial of intraarterial treatment for acute ischemic stroke. N Engl J Med. 2015;372(1):11–20.

108. Molina CA, Chamorro A, Rovira A, de Miquel A, Serena J, Roman LS, et al. REVASCAT: a randomized trial of revascularization with SOLITAIRE FR device vs. best medical therapy in the treatment of acute stroke due to anterior circulation large vessel occlusion presenting within eight-hours of symptom onset. Int J Stroke. 2015;10(4):619–26.
109. Bracard SP, Ducrocq XP, Mas JLP, Soudant MMS, Oppenheim CP, Moulin TP, et al. Mechanical thrombectomy after intravenous alteplase versus alteplase alone after stroke (THRACE): a randomised controlled trial. Lancet Neurol. 2016;15(11):1138–47.
110. Goyal M, Menon BK, van Zwam WH, Dippel DW, Mitchell PJ, Demchuk AM, et al. Endovascular thrombectomy after large-vessel ischaemic stroke: a meta-analysis of individual patient data from five randomised trials. Lancet. 2016;387(10029):1723–31.
111. Mokin M, Ansari SA, McTaggart RA, Bulsara KR, Goyal M, Chen M, et al. Indications for thrombectomy in acute ischemic stroke from emergent large vessel occlusion (ELVO): report of the SNIS Standards and Guidelines Committee. J Neurointerv Surg. 2019;11(3):215–20.
112. Cagnazzo F, Derraz I, Dargazanli C, Lefevre P-H, Gascou G, Riquelme C, et al. Mechanical thrombectomy in patients with acute ischemic stroke and ASPECTS ≤6: a meta-analysis. J Neurointerv Surg. 2020;12(4):350–5.
113. Katsanos AH, Catanese L, Shoamanesh A. Endovascular thrombectomy in patients with very low ASPECTS scores: a systematic review and meta-analysis. Neurology. 2023;101(20):e2043–e5.
114. Chen L, Deng YS, Wang LY, Mao XQ, Zhang C, Liu ZT, et al. Successful endovascular thrombectomy using Solitaire FR stent with intermediate catheter assisting technique for acute persistent primitive trigeminal artery and basilar artery occlusion: a case report and literature review. Surg Neurol Int. 2024;15:93.
115. Bao L, Liu Y, Chen L, Wang F, Zhu Y, Liang S, et al. Effects of Solitaire AB stent thrombectomy with tirofiban and butylphthalide on neurological function and inflammatory factors in acute cerebral infarction patients. Int J Neurosci. 2024;1-10:1.
116. Zaidat OO, Ikeme S, Sheth SA, Yoshimura S, Yang XG, Brinjikji W, et al. MASTRO I: meta-analysis and systematic review of thrombectomy stent retriever outcomes: comparing functional, safety and recanalization outcomes between EmboTrap, Solitaire and Trevo in acute ischemic stroke. J Comp Eff Res. 2023;12(5):e230001.
117. Ntoulias N, Brehm A, Tsogkas I, Jesser J, Caragliano AA, Demerath T, et al. Initial experience with the Solitaire X 3 mm stent retriever for the treatment of distal medium vessel occlusions. J Clin Med. 2023;12(23):7289.
118. Luo G, Yan X, Xiao G, Wei L, Nai Bi Jiang YLK, Ma R, et al. Comparing a novel Catfish flow restoration device and the Solitaire stent retriever for thrombectomy revascularisation in emergent large vessel occlusion stroke: a prospective randomised controlled study. Stroke Vasc Neurol. 2023;8(6):435–43.
119. Biederko R, Honig A, Shabad K, Zlotnik Y, Ben-Arie G, Alguayn F, et al. Improved first-pass effect in acute stroke thrombectomy using Solitaire-X compared to Solitaire-FR. Front Neurol. 2023;14:1215349.
120. Zhou T, Li T, Zhu L, Li Z, Li Q, Bai WX, et al. Comparing the efficacy and safety of the Skyflow device with those of the Solitaire FR stent in patients with acute ischemic stroke: a prospective, multicenter, randomized, non-inferiority clinical trial. J Neurointerv Surg. 2022;14(11):1130–4.
121. Wang T, Dong S, Zhang M, Yu C, Xue M, Chen A. Effect of Solitaire FR stent thrombectomy combined with the suction thrombus on the clinical effect and prognosis of acute middle cerebral artery occlusion. Evid Based Complement Alternat Med. 2022;2022:9227790.
122. Fischer U, Kaesmacher J, Plattner PS, Butikofer L, Mordasini P, Deppeler S, et al. SWIFT DIRECT: Solitaire with the intention for thrombectomy plus intravenous t-PA versus DIRECT Solitaire stent-retriever thrombectomy in acute anterior circulation stroke: methodology of a randomized, controlled, multicentre study. Int J Stroke. 2022;17(6):698–705.
123. Oliver MJ, Brereton E, Khan MA, Davis A, Singer J. Trevo 6 x 25mm vs. 4 x 30mm in mechanical thrombectomy of M1 LVO. Front Neurol. 2021;12:677630.

124. Jadhav AP, Desai SM, Budzik RF, Gupta R, Baxter B, English JD, et al. First pass effect in patients with large vessel occlusion strokes undergoing neurothrombectomy: insights from the Trevo Retriever Registry. J Neurointerv Surg. 2021;13(7):619–22.
125. Etter MM, Mohlenbruch M, Weyland CS, Perez-Garcia C, Moreu M, Capasso F, et al. Initial experience with the Trevo NXT stent retriever. Front Neurol. 2021;12:704329.
126. Kim SH, Lee H, Kim SB, Kim ST, Baek JW, Heo YJ, et al. Hybrid mechanical thrombectomy for acute ischemic stroke using an intermediate aspiration catheter and Trevo stent simultaneously. J Clin Neurosci. 2020;76:9–14.
127. Nogueira RG, Haussen DC, Castonguay A, Rebello LC, Abraham M, Puri A, et al. Site experience and outcomes in the Trevo Acute Ischemic Stroke (TRACK) Multicenter Registry. Stroke. 2019;50(9):2455–60.
128. Yi HJ, Lee DH, Kim SU. Effectiveness of Trevo stent retriever in acute ischemic stroke: comparison with Solitaire stent. Medicine (Baltimore). 2018;97(20):e10747.
129. Imahori T, Okamura Y, Sakata J, Shose H, Yokote A, Matsushima K, et al. Stent expansion and in-stent thrombus sign in the Trevo stent retriever predict recanalization and possible etiology during mechanical thrombectomy: a case series of 50 patients with acute middle cerebral artery occlusion. World Neurosurg. 2018;124:e303.
130. Binning MJ, Bartolini B, Baxter B, Budzik R, English J, Gupta R, et al. Trevo 2000: results of a large real-world registry for stent retriever for acute ischemic stroke. J Am Heart Assoc. 2018;7(24):e010867.
131. Kabbasch C, Mpotsaris A, Liebig T, Soderman M, Holtmannspotter M, Cronqvist M, et al. First-in-man procedural experience with the novel EmboTrap(R) revascularization device for the treatment of ischemic stroke-a European multicenter series. Clin Neuroradiol. 2016;26(2):221–8.
132. Bourcier R, Abed D, Piotin M, Redjem H, Ferre JC, Eugene F, et al. Multicenter initial experience with the EmboTrap device in acute anterior ischemic stroke. J Neuroradiol. 2018;45(4):230–5.
133. Zaidat OO, Bozorgchami H, Ribo M, Saver JL, Mattle HP, Chapot R, et al. Primary results of the multicenter ARISE II study (analysis of revascularization in ischemic stroke with EmboTrap). Stroke. 2018;49(5):1107–15.
134. Valente I, Nappini S, Renieri L, Pedicelli A, Lozupone E, Colosimo C, et al. Initial experience with the novel EmboTrap II clot-retrieving device for the treatment of ischaemic stroke. Interv Neuroradiol. 2019;25(3):271–6.
135. Baek JH, Kim BM, Suh SH, Jeon HJ, Ihm EH, Park H, et al. First-Pass Recanalization with EmboTrap II in Acute Ischemic Stroke (FREE-AIS): a multicenter prospective study. Korean J Radiol. 2023;24(2):145–54.
136. Namitome S, Nagao Y, Shigehatake Y, Matsuo J, Kawamoto K, Kuroki K, et al. Evaluation of partial resheathing of EmboTrap III using the microcatheter (PREMIER) technique for fibrin-rich hard clots in an in vitro vessel model. Front Neurol. 2024;15:1368890.
137. Becker KJ, Brott TG. Approval of the MERCI clot retriever: a critical view. Stroke. 2005;36(2):400–3.
138. Pérez MA, Miloslavski E, Fischer S, Bäzner H, Henkes H. Intracranial thrombectomy using the Solitaire stent: a historical vignette. J Neurointerv Surg. 2012;4(6):e32.
139. Nogueira RG, Lobsien D, Klisch J, Pielenz D, Lobsien E, Sauvageau E, et al. Thrombectomy with the pRESET vs Solitaire stent retrievers as first-line large vessel occlusion stroke treatment: a randomized clinical trial. JAMA Neurol. 2024;81(2):170–8.
140. Baek JW, Heo YJ, Kim ST, Seo JH, Jeong HW, Kim EG. Comparison of the Solitaire and Trevo stents for endovascular treatment of acute ischemic stroke: a single. Center experience. Neurol India. 2021;69(2):378–82.
141. Liang CW, Toor HJ, Duran Martinez E, Sheth SA, Chao K, Feng L, et al. First pass recanalization rates of Solitaire vs Trevo vs primary aspiration: the Kaiser Southern California experience. Perm J. 2020;25:1–3.

142. Ntoulias N, Brehm A, Miralbes S, Naravetla B, Spiotta A, Loehr C, et al. Trevo 3 Mm and/or AXS catalyst 5 for the treatment of medium distal vessel occlusion stroke-results from the ASSIST Registry. Clin Neuroradiol. 2024; https://doi.org/10.1007/s00062-024-01450-y.
143. Zhao CH, Koneru M, Siegler JE, Vigilante N, Khalife J, Tonetti DA, et al. Single center experience using 3 mm Trevo stent retrievers in medium vessel occlusion thrombectomy. Interv Neuroradiol. 2023; https://doi.org/10.1177/15910199231199880.
144. Zhang X, Liu J, Han H, Zhang P, Chen X, Yuan H, et al. Effectiveness and safety of the Trevo(R) retriever for mechanical thrombectomy in Chinese patients with acute ischemic stroke: Trevo Retriever China Registry. Interv Neuroradiol. 2023; https://doi.org/10.1177/15910199231151275.
145. Uchida K, Sakai N, Yamagami H, Uemura K, Imamura H, Takeuchi M, et al. Japan Trevo Registry: real-world registry of stent retriever alone or in combined therapy with aspiration catheter for acute ischemic stroke in Japan. Neurol Med Chir (Tokyo). 2023;63(11):503–11.
146. Yi HJ, Lee DH, Sung JH. Comparison of FlowGate(2) and Merci as balloon guide catheters used in mechanical thrombectomies for stroke intervention. Exp Ther Med. 2020;20(2):1129–36.
147. Mokin M, Primiani CT, Castonguay AC, Nogueira RG, Haussen DC, English JD, et al. First pass effect in patients treated with the Trevo stent-retriever: a TRACK registry study analysis. Front Neurol. 2020;11:83.
148. Haussen DC, Eby B, Al-Bayati AR, Grossberg JA, Rodrigues GM, Frankel MR, et al. A comparative analysis of 3MAX aspiration versus 3 mm Trevo Retriever for distal occlusion thrombectomy in acute stroke. J Neurointerv Surg. 2020;12(3):279–82.
149. Brinjikji W, Starke RM, Murad MH, Fiorella D, Pereira VM, Goyal M, et al. Impact of balloon guide catheter on technical and clinical outcomes: a systematic review and meta-analysis. J Neurointerv Surg. 2018;10(4):335–9.
150. Chueh JY, Marosfoi MG, Brooks OW, King RM, Puri AS, Gounis MJ. Novel distal emboli protection technology: the EmboTrap. Interv Neurol. 2017;6(3–4):268–76.
151. Hamada Y, Matsuoka H, Sato S, Kawabata Y, Iwamoto K, Ikeda M, et al. Combining the deployment of only the distal basket segment of the EMBOTRAP III and an aspiration catheter for M2 occlusions: the ONE-SEG technique. Front Neurol. 2024;15:1424030.
152. Siddiqui AH, Waqas M, Brinjikji W, De Meyer SF, Doyle K, Fiehler J, et al. Embotrap Extraction & Clot Evaluation & Lesion Evaluation for NeuroThrombectomy (EXCELLENT) Registry design and methods. J Neurointerv Surg. 2022;14(8):783–7.
153. Siddiqui AH, Waqas M, Andersson T, Saver JL, Mattle HP, Bozorgchami H, et al. Predictors of unfavorable outcomes despite substantial reperfusion: insights from analysis of revascularization in ischemic stroke with EmboTrap II study. Interv Neuroradiol. 2022;28(5):556–61.
154. Brinjikji W, Ikeme S, Kottenmeier E, Khaled A, M S, Khanna R. Real-world outcomes associated with the use of the EmboTrap revascularization device for ischemic stroke in the United States. J Neurointerv Surg. 2022;14(11):1068–72.
155. Bala F, Ferrigno M, Personnic T, Estrade L, Karam A, Henon H, et al. Thrombectomy using the EmboTrap II device in late treatment patients in the real-world setting. World Neurosurg. 2021;151:e387–e94.
156. Brehm A, Maus V, Tsogkas I, Colla R, Hesse AC, Gera RG, et al. Stent-retriever assisted vacuum-locked extraction (SAVE) versus a direct aspiration first pass technique (ADAPT) for acute stroke: data from the real-world. BMC Neurol. 2019;19(1):65.
157. Benndorf G, Bender A, Lehmann R, Lanksch W. Transvenous occlusion of dural cavernous sinus fistulas through the thrombosed inferior petrosal sinus: report of four cases and review of the literature. Surg Neurol. 2000;54(1):42–54.
158. Adusumilli G, Kobeissi H, Ghozy S, Kallmes KM, Brinjikji W, Kallmes DF, et al. Comparing Tigertriever 13 to other thrombectomy devices for distal medium vessel occlusion: a systematic review and meta-analysis. Interv Neuroradiol. 2023; https://doi.org/10.1177/15910199231152510.

159. Fischer S, Will L, Phung T, Weber W, Maus V, Nordmeyer H. The Tigertriever 13 for mechanical thrombectomy in distal and medium intracranial vessel occlusions. Neuroradiology. 2022;64(4):775–83.
160. Ojeda DJ, Ghannam M, Sanchez S, Almajali M, Koul P, Saver JL, et al. Tigertriever in the treatment of acute ischemic stroke with underlying intracranial atherosclerotic disease. J Neurointerv Surg. 2024;16(11):1083–7.
161. Piasecki P, Wierzbicki M, Narloch J, Debiec A, Staszewski J. Mechanical thrombectomy of large vessel occlusion using adjustable vs. self-expanding stent-retriever-comparison of Tigertriever device with stent-like stent-retrievers: a propensity score analysis. Front Neurol. 2022;13:1032307.
162. Will L, Maus V, Maurer C, Weber A, Weber W, Fischer S. Mechanical thrombectomy in acute ischemic stroke using a manually expandable stent retriever (Tigertriever): preliminary single center experience. Clin Neuroradiol. 2021;31(2):491–7.
163. Piasecki P, Wierzbicki M, Narloch J. Safety and efficacy of mechanical thrombectomy using Tigertriever as a rescue device after failed aspiration-single center experience. Front Neurol. 2020;11:603679.
164. Gruber P, Diepers M, von Hessling A, Weber J, Kahles T, Anon J, et al. Mechanical thrombectomy using the new Tigertriever in acute ischemic stroke patients—a Swiss prospective multicenter study. Interv Neuroradiol. 2020;26(5):598–601.
165. Kara B, Selcuk HH, Yildiz O, Cetinkaya D. Revascularization of acute basilar artery occlusion using the Tigertriever adjustable clot retriever. Clin Neuroradiol. 2017;27(2):241–3.
166. Turk AS, Spiotta A, Frei D, Mocco J, Baxter B, Fiorella D, et al. Initial clinical experience with the ADAPT technique: a direct aspiration first pass technique for stroke thrombectomy. J Neurointerv Surg. 2014;6(3):231–7.
167. Molinaro S, Russo R, Mistretta F, Risi G, Bergui M. Maximizing the available space : the new RED 062 aspiration catheter in conjunction with 7F guide catheter in mechanical thrombectomy for left anterior circulation stroke via direct transradial approach. Clin Neuroradiol. 2023;33(3):865–8.
168. Requena M, Pinana C, Olive-Gadea M, Hernandez D, Boned S, De Dios M, et al. Combined technique as first approach in mechanical thrombectomy: efficacy and safety of REACT catheter combined with stent retriever. Interv Neuroradiol. 2023;29(5):504–9.
169. Sundar K, Paulraj S, Choudhury SR, Hassan H, Sengupta J, Pattari SK. Successful endovascular treatment of cerebral venous thrombosis with a novel, larger aspiration catheter (REACT): a case report. Neurointervention. 2021;16(1):83–7.
170. Raymond SB, Nasir-Moin M, Koch MJ, Rabinov JD, Leslie-Mazwi T, Patel AB. Initial experience with React 68 aspiration catheter. Interv Neuroradiol. 2020;26(3):358–63.
171. Akmangit I, Sayin B, Karaman A, Daglioglu E, Arli B, Sahin MH, et al. Endovascular stroke therapy focused on direct clot aspiration using the SOFIA(TM) catheter for acute ischemic stroke. Turk Neurosurg. 2022;32(5):720–6.
172. Bolognini F, Lebedinsky PA, Musacchio M, Delaitre M, Traore AM, Vuillemet F, et al. SOFIA catheter for direct aspiration of large vessel occlusion stroke: a single-center cohort and meta-analysis. Interv Neuroradiol. 2021;27(6):850–7.
173. Bilgin C, Durmus Y, Haki C, Nas OF, Hakyemez B. Direct aspiration thrombectomy experience with the SOFIA 6F catheter in acute ischemic stroke. Jpn J Radiol. 2021;39(6):605–10.
174. Heit JJ, et al. Correction: Sofia intermediate catheter and the SNAKE technique: safety and efficacy of the Sofia catheter without guidewire or microcatheter construct. J Neurointerv Surg. 2021;13(6):e12.
175. Wessell AP, Cannarsa G, Carvalho H, Kole MJ, Sharma P, Le EJ, et al. Thrombectomy for acute ischemic stroke with the new Sofia 6-French PLUS distal access reperfusion catheter: a single-center experience. Neuroradiol J. 2020;33(1):17–23.
176. Oguz S, Dinc H, Ozturk MH. A back and forth manual aspiration technique using a SOFIA Plus catheter for acute ischemic stroke: technical note. Neuroradiology. 2019;61(1):109–11.

177. Nouri N, Ferrigno M, Personnic T, Bala F, Bretzner M, Estrade L, et al. Real-world thrombectomy using the Sofia catheter. World Neurosurg. 2019;122:e1247–e51.
178. Li H, Liu JF, Li CH, Wang JW, Tian YY. Successful thrombectomy using Sofia (6F) PLUS catheter in acute stroke patient with coincident proximal unruptured aneurysm. World Neurosurg. 2019;132:245–50.
179. Kim YW, Hwang YH, Kim YS, Kang DH. Frontline contact aspiration thrombectomy using SOFIA catheter for acute ischemic stroke: period-to-period comparison with Penumbra catheter. Acta Neurochir. 2019;161(6):1197–204.
180. Shallwani H, Shakir HJ, Rangel-Castilla L, Davies JM, Sonig A, Sattur MG, et al. Safety and efficacy of the Sofia (6F) PLUS distal access reperfusion catheter in the endovascular treatment of acute ischemic stroke. Neurosurgery. 2018;82(3):312–21.
181. Heit JJ, Wong JH, Mofaff AM, Telischak NA, Dodd RL, Marks MP, et al. Sofia intermediate catheter and the SNAKE technique: safety and efficacy of the Sofia catheter without guidewire or microcatheter construct. J Neurointerv Surg. 2018;10(4):401–6.
182. Wong JHY, Do HM, Telischak NA, Moraff AM, Dodd RL, Marks MP, et al. Initial experience with SOFIA as an intermediate catheter in mechanical thrombectomy for acute ischemic stroke. J Neurointerv Surg. 2017;9(11):1103–6.
183. Mohlenbruch MA, Kabbasch C, Kowoll A, Broussalis E, Sonnberger M, Muller M, et al. Multicenter experience with the new SOFIA Plus catheter as a primary local aspiration catheter for acute stroke thrombectomy. J Neurointerv Surg. 2017;9(12):1223–7.
184. Kabbasch C, Mohlenbruch M, Stampfl S, Mpotsaris A, Behme D, Liebig T. First-line lesional aspiration in acute stroke thrombectomy using a novel intermediate catheter: initial experiences with the SOFIA. Interv Neuroradiol. 2016;22(3):333–9.
185. Schramm P, Navia P, Papa R, Zamarro J, Tomasello A, Weber W, et al. ADAPT technique with ACE68 and ACE64 reperfusion catheters in ischemic stroke treatment: results from the PROMISE study. J Neurointerv Surg. 2019;11(3):226–31.
186. Frölich AM, Kim W, Stribrny K, Jansen O, Möhlenbruch M, Szikora I, et al. The novel Tenzing 7 delivery catheter designed to deliver intermediate catheters to the face of embolus without crossing: clinical performance predicted in anatomically challenging model. J Neurointerv Surg. 2021;13(8):722.
187. Settecase F, Kim WT, Sivapatham T, Khangura R, Caldwell J, Lee S, et al. Improved catheter delivery for aspiration thrombectomy using Tenzing 7 ledge reducing catheter and FreeClimb 70. Interv Neuroradiol. 2023; https://doi.org/10.1177/15910199231177754.
188. Yaeger K, Iserson A, Singh P, Wolf J, Vidal E, Oxley T, et al. A technical comparison of thrombectomy vacuum aspiration systems. J Neurointerv Surg. 2020;12(1):72–6.
189. Turk AS 3rd, Siddiqui A, Fifi JT, De Leacy RA, Fiorella DJ, Gu E, et al. Aspiration thrombectomy versus stent retriever thrombectomy as first-line approach for large vessel occlusion (COMPASS): a multicentre, randomised, open label, blinded outcome, non-inferiority trial. Lancet. 2019;393(10175):998–1008.
190. Mokin M, Waqas M, Fifi J, De Leacy R, Fiorella D, Levy EI, et al. Clot perviousness is associated with first pass success of aspiration thrombectomy in the COMPASS trial. J Neurointerv Surg. 2021;13(6):509–14.
191. Lan X, Liang Z, Shen C, Yi W, Ni F, Zhang Z, et al. Endovascular treatment of embolism-related acute basilar artery occlusion stroke: ADAPT versus stent retriever thrombectomy. Interv Neuroradiol. 2024; https://doi.org/10.1177/15910199241254137.
192. Peschillo S, Tomasello A, Diana F, Hernandez D, Toccaceli G, Rosal-Fontana M, et al. Comparison of subacute vascular damage caused by ADAPT versus stent retriever devices after thrombectomy in acute ischemic stroke: histological and ultrastructural study in an animal model. Interv Neurol. 2018;7(6):501–12.
193. Choi JW, Han M, Park JH, Jung WS. Effect of manual aspiration thrombectomy using large-bore aspiration catheter for acute basilar artery occlusion: comparison with a stent retriever system. BMC Neurol. 2020;20(1):434.

194. Peschillo S, Diana F, Berge J, Missori P. A comparison of acute vascular damage caused by ADAPT versus a stent retriever device after thrombectomy in acute ischemic stroke: a histological and ultrastructural study in an animal model. J Neurointerv Surg. 2017;9(8):743–9.
195. Pampana E, Fabiano S, De Rubeis G, Bertaccini L, Stasolla A, Pingi A, et al. Switch strategy from direct aspiration first pass technique to Solumbra improves technical outcome in endovascularly treated stroke. Int J Environ Res Public Health. 2021;18(5):2670.
196. Jablonska M, Li J, Tiberi R, Canals P, Ortega S, Tomasello A, et al. Partial (SAVE) versus complete (Solumbra) stent retriever retraction technique for mechanical thrombectomy: a randomized in vitro study. AJNR Am J Neuroradiol. 2023;44(10):1165–70.
197. Ezzeldin M, Ota R, Riha E, Delora A, Alenzi B, Gordon V, et al. Use of angled-tip aspiration catheters is associated with a lower cost of thrombectomy in patients with acute ischemic stroke secondary to large and medium vessel occlusions. Interv Neuroradiol. 2023; https://doi.org/10.1177/15910199231198914.
198. Nogueira RG, Geyik S, Bajrami A, Erdem E, Ertugrul OZ, Montalverne FJ, et al. Abstract WMP96: a prospective trial of the Rapidpulse Tm aspiration system as frontline approach for stroke thrombectomy (RapidPulseFS). Stroke (1970). 2023;54(Suppl_1) https://doi.org/10.1161/str.54.suppl_1.WMP96.
199. Venketasubramanian N, Yeo LLL, Tan B, Chan BPL. Sonothrombolysis for ischemic stroke. J Cardiovasc Dev Dis. 2024;11(3):75.
200. Jiang Z, Jiang N, Wang Z, Deng Q, Zhou Q, Hu B. Ultrasound-mediated cardiovascular thrombolysis: from Sonothrombolysis to Sonoperfusion. Postgrad Med J. 2024; https://doi.org/10.1093/postmj/qgae127.
201. George Mathen P, Krupa J, Samson N, Mirza S, Raja H, Selvaraj S, et al. Safety, feasibility and efficacy of sonothrombolysis with micro boluses of perfluoropropane as a point of care therapy for patients with acute ST-elevation myocardial infarction. J R Coll Physicians Edinb. 2024;54(3):197–203.
202. Brinjikji W, Kottenmeier E, Kabiri M, Khaled A, Pederson JM, Al-Bayati AR. Estimating the impact of balloon guide catheter with mechanical thrombectomy for acute ischemic stroke: a U.S. cost analysis. Interv Neuroradiol. 2023; https://doi.org/10.1177/15910199231191034.
203. Dossani RH, Waqas M, Rai HH, Monteiro A, Almayman F, Cappuzzo JM, et al. Use of Walrus balloon-guide catheter through sheathless radial approach for mechanical thrombectomy of right middle cerebral artery occlusion. J Neurointerv Surg. 2022;14(5):521.
204. Kang BM, Yi HJ, Shin DS, Kim BT. Effect of early balloon inflation of balloon guide catheter in mechanical thrombectomy for large vessel occlusion. Curr Neurovasc Res. 2023;20(1):124–31.
205. Lee IH, Ha SK, Lim DJ, Choi JI. Distal placement of balloon guide catheter facilitates stent-retriever mechanical thrombectomy for acute ischemic stroke in the anterior circulation. Acta Neurochir. 2023;165(12):3759–68.
206. Podlasek A, Dhillon PS, Jewett G, Shahein A, Goyal M, Almekhlafi M. Clinical and procedural outcomes with or without balloon guide catheters during endovascular thrombectomy in acute ischemic stroke: a systematic review and meta-analysis with first-line technique subgroup analysis. AJNR Am J Neuroradiol. 2021;42(8):1464–71.
207. Terceno M, Bashir S, Puig J, Daunis-I-Estadella J, Murias E, Jimenez JM, et al. Impact of balloon guide catheters in elderly patients treated with mechanical thrombectomy: insights from the ROSSETTI Registry. AJNR Am J Neuroradiol. 2023;44(11):1275–81.
208. Topiwala K, Quinn C, Mehta T, Masood K, Grande A, Tummala R, et al. BOBBY balloon guide catheter thrombectomy in large-vessel occlusion stroke: initial experience. Interv Neuroradiol. 2024;30(1):80–5.
209. Velasco A, Buerke B, Stracke CP, Berkemeyer S, Mosimann PJ, Schwindt W, et al. Comparison of a balloon guide catheter and a non-balloon guide catheter for mechanical thrombectomy. Radiology. 2016;280(1):169–76.

210. Orscelik A, Kallmes DF, Bilgin C, Musmar B, Senol YC, Kobeissi H, et al. Comparison of balloon guide catheter versus non-balloon guide catheter for mechanical thrombectomy in patients with distal medium vessel occlusion. J Neurointerv Surg. 2024;16(6):587–94.
211. Nguyen TN, Castonguay AC, Nogueira RG, Haussen DC, English JD, Satti SR, et al. Effect of balloon guide catheter on clinical outcomes and reperfusion in Trevo thrombectomy. J Neurointerv Surg. 2019;11(9):861–5.
212. Gravino G, Jakobek W, Nayak S, Yang Y, Ranjbar J, Roffe C. Correspondence on 'Comparison of balloon guide catheter versus non-balloon guide catheter for mechanical thrombectomy in patients with distal medium vessel occlusion' by Orscelik et al. J Neurointerv Surg. 2024;16(6):631–2.
213. Cappuzzo JM, Monteiro A, Waqas M, Baig AA, Popoola DO, Almayman F, et al. Carotid artery stenting using the Walrus balloon guide catheter with flow reversal for proximal embolic protection: technical description and single-center case series. Oper Neurosurg (Hagerstown, Md). 2023;24(1):11–6.
214. Forman J, Ricotta JJ, Ricotta JJ. "TCAR or nothing": the only options for some complex carotid stenosis. J Vasc Surg Cases Innov Tech. 2024;10(2):101404.
215. AbuRahma AF, Avgerinos ED, Chang RW, Darling RC, Duncan AA, Forbes TL, et al. The Society for Vascular Surgery implementation document for management of extracranial cerebrovascular disease. J Vasc Surg. 2022;75(1, Supplement):26S–98S.
216. Delvoye F, Maier B, Escalard S, Labreuche J, Thion LA, Aknouche S, et al. Antiplatelet therapy during emergent extracranial internal carotid artery stenting: comparison of three intravenous antiplatelet perioperative strategies. J Stroke Cerebrovasc Dis. 2021;30(2):105521.
217. Sussman ES, Jin M, Pendharkar AV, Pulli B, Feng A, Heit JJ, et al. Dual antiplatelet therapy after carotid artery stenting: trends and outcomes in a large national database. J Neurointerv Surg. 2021;13(1):8–13.
218. Pomero F, Galli E, Bellesini M, Maroni L, Squizzato A. P2Y12 inhibitors plus aspirin for acute treatment and secondary prevention in minor stroke and high-risk transient ischemic attack: a systematic review and meta-analysis. Eur J Intern Med. 2022;100:46–55.
219. Savi P, Nurden P, Nurden AT, Levy-Toledano S, Herbert JM. Clopidogrel: a review of its mechanism of action. Platelets. 1998;9(3–4):251–5.
220. Marcaccio CL, Patel PB, Liang P, Rastogi V, Stangenberg L, Jim J, et al. Efficacy and safety of perioperative dual antiplatelet therapy with ticagrelor versus clopidogrel in carotid artery stenting. J Vasc Surg. 2022;75(4):1293–303 e8.
221. Mazzaccaro D, Giannetta M, Ranucci M, Righini P, Di Dedda U, Baryshnikova E, et al. Clopidogrel resistance and ticagrelor replacement in dual antiplatelet therapy for carotid artery stenting. Ann Vasc Surg. 2023;90:128–36.
222. Pandya D, Fitzsimmons B, Wolfe T, Hussain S, Lynch J, Ortega-Gutierrez S, et al. Measurement of antiplatelet inhibition during neurointerventional procedures: the effect of antithrombotic duration and loading dose. J Neuroimaging. 2010;20(1):64–9.
223. Sorkin GC, Dumont TM, Wach MM, Eller JL, Mokin M, Natarajan SK, et al. Carotid artery stenting outcomes: do they correlate with antiplatelet response assays? J Neurointerv Surg. 2014;6(5):373.
224. Song T-J, Suh SH, Min P-K, Kim DJ, Kim BM, Heo JH, et al. The influence of anti-platelet resistance on the development of cerebral ischemic lesion after carotid artery stenting. Yonsei Med J. 2013;54(2):288–94.
225. Muram S, Panchendrabose K, Eagles ME, Salam MSA, Eesa M, Agbani EO, et al. Natural history of antiplatelet nonresponders undergoing carotid artery stenting. J Neurosurg. 2023;139(3):661–9.
226. Mazzaccaro D, Ranucci M, Nano G. Clopidogrel resistance in dual antiplatelet therapy after carotid stenting. J Vasc Surg. 2021;74(6):2119.
227. Mousa SA, Jeske WP, Fareed J. Antiplatelet therapy prasugrel: a novel platelet ADP P2Y12 receptor antagonist. Clin Appl Thromb Hemost. 2010;16(2):170–6.

228. Angiolillo DJ, Suryadevara S, Capranzano P, Bass TA. Prasugrel: a novel platelet ADP P2Y12 receptor antagonist. A review on its mechanism of action and clinical development. Expert Opin Pharmacother. 2008;9(16):2893–900.
229. Floyd J, Wolfe S. Prasugrel STEMI subgroup analysis. Lancet (Br Ed). 2009;373(9678):1845–6.
230. Cattaneo M. New $P2Y_{12}$ inhibitors. Circulation. 2010;121(1):171–9.
231. Birkeland K, Parra D, Rosenstein R. Antiplatelet therapy in acute coronary syndromes: focus on ticagrelor. J Blood Med. 2010;1(1):197–219.
232. Pop R, Finitsis SN, Marnat G, Derraz I, Cognard C, Calviere L, et al. Cangrelor for emergent carotid stenting during stroke thrombectomy: a comparative analysis versus glycoprotein IIb/IIIa inhibitors or aspirin monotherapy. J Neurointerv Surg. 2024; https://doi.org/10.1136/jnis-2024-022125.
233. Waldron NH, Dallas T, Erhunmwunsee L, Wang TY, Berry MF, Welsby IJ. Bleeding risk associated with eptifibatide (Integrilin) bridging in thoracic surgery patients. J Thromb Thrombolysis. 2017;43(2):194–202.
234. Pop R, Severac F, Hasiu A, Mihoc D, Mangin PH, Chibbaro S, et al. Conservative versus aggressive antiplatelet strategy for emergent carotid stenting during stroke thrombectomy. Interv Neuroradiol. 2022;29(3):268–76.
235. Viglas P, Smolka V, Raupach J, Hejcl A, Cernik D, Cihlar F. Outcome of tailored antiplatelet therapy in carotid stenting: a retrospective comparative study. CVIR Endovasc. 2024;7(1):73.
236. Milazzo N, Da Ros V, Diomedi M, Menozzi R, Pezzini A, Ruggiero M, et al. Current trends in antiplatelet strategies for emergent carotid stenting in acute tandem occlusions: a web-based, nationwide survey in the Italian neurovascular community. Neurol Sci. 2024; https://doi.org/10.1007/s10072-024-07722-2.
237. De Rubeis G, Prosperini L, Badia S, Fabiano S, Bertaccini L, Wlderk A, et al. Profile of antiplatelet regimens for emergent carotid stenting in tandem occlusion. Systematic review and meta-analysis. Clin Neurol Neurosurg. 2024;247:108595.
238. Pop R, Severac F, Hasiu A, Mihoc D, Mangin PH, Chibbaro S, et al. Conservative versus aggressive antiplatelet strategy for emergent carotid stenting during stroke thrombectomy. Interv Neuroradiol. 2023;29(3):268–76.
239. Marnat G, Finistis S, Moreno R, Sibon I, Pop R, Mazighi M, et al. Aspirin versus aggressive antiplatelet therapy for acute carotid stenting plus thrombectomy in tandem occlusions: ETIS Registry results. J Neurointerv Surg. 2023;15(e2):e248–e54.
240. Pop R, Hasiu A, Mangin PH, Severac F, Mihoc D, Nistoran D, et al. Postprocedural antiplatelet treatment after emergent carotid stenting in tandem lesions stroke: impact on stent patency beyond day 1. AJNR Am J Neuroradiol. 2021;42(5):921–5.
241. Hadler F, Singh R, Wiesmann M, Reich A, Nikoubashman O. Increased rates of hemorrhages after endovascular stroke treatment with emergency carotid artery stenting and dual antiplatelet therapy. Cerebrovasc Dis. 2021;50(2):162–70.
242. Goyal M, Yoshimura S, Milot G, Fiehler J, Jayaraman M, Dorn F, et al. Considerations for antiplatelet management of carotid stenting in the setting of mechanical Thrombectomy: a Delphi consensus statement. AJNR Am J Neuroradiol. 2020;41(12):2274–9.
243. Qureshi AI, Jahngir MU, Qualls K, Akinci Y, Lobanova I, Liaqat J, et al. The effect of ticagrelor on platelet reactivity in patients with clopidogrel resistance undergoing neuroendovascular procedures. J Neuroimaging. 2020;30(3):327–34.
244. Faught RWF, Satti SR, Hurst RW, Pukenas BA, Smith MJ. Heterogeneous practice patterns regarding antiplatelet medications for neuroendovascular stenting in the USA: a multicenter survey. J Neurointerv Surg. 2014;6(10):774.
245. Vatan MB, Acar BA, Aksoy M, Can Y, Varim C, Agac MT, et al. Predictors of periprocedural complications of carotid artery stenting—a multivariate analysis of a single-centre experience. Vasa. 2016;45(5):387–93.
246. Fanous AA, Jowdy PK, Morr S, Vakharia K, Shallwani H, Lorincz K, et al. Vascular anatomy and not age is responsible for increased risk of complications in symptomatic elderly patients undergoing carotid artery stenting. World Neurosurg. 2019;128:e513–e21.

247. Kim NY, Choi JW, Whang K, Cho SM, Koo YM, Kim JY. Neurologic complications in patients with carotid artery stenting. J Cerebrovasc Endovasc Neurosurg. 2019;21(2):86–93.
248. Low M, Gray BH, Dicks AB, Ochiobi O, Blas JVV, Gandhi SS, et al. Comparison of complications and cost for transfemoral versus transcarotid stenting of carotid artery stenosis. Ann Vasc Surg. 2023;89:1–10.
249. Muszynski P, Richard S, Finitsis S, Humbertjean L, Audibert G, Mione G, et al. Transradial access with Simmons guiding catheter for carotid artery stenting: feasibility and procedural complications in a single-center experience. Interv Neuroradiol. 2023; https://doi.org/10.1177/15910199231171845.
250. Ozaki S, Akimoto T, Iida Y, Miyake S, Suzuki R, Shimohigoshi W, et al. Complications and outcomes of carotid artery stenting in high-risk cases. J Stroke Cerebrovasc Dis. 2023;32(10):107329.
251. Ozdemir M, Sevinc OF. Relationship between carotid artery stenosis percentage and complications in patients treated with carotid stenting. Eur Rev Med Pharmacol Sci. 2024;28(8):3263–7.
252. Tahtabasi M, Camurcuoglu E, Erdem U, Ozdemir AS, Kaya V. Carotid artery stenting in unfavorable vascular anatomy: effect of embolic protection filter use on periprocedural complications. J Clin Neurosci. 2024;128:110787.
253. Almenoff M, Garrett HE Jr. Evaluation of staged TCAR and cardiac surgery or structural heart intervention. Vasc Endovasc Surg. 2021;55(7):702–5.
254. Beeman BR, Kuhn BA, Recht MH, Muck PE, Schneider PA. Duplex ultrasound surveillance after Transcarotid Artery Revascularization (TCAR) in clinical practice. Ann Vasc Surg. 2021;72:330–9.
255. Dakour-Aridi H, Ramakrishnan G, Zarrintan S, Malas MB. Outcomes of transcarotid revascularization with dynamic flow reversal versus carotid endarterectomy in the TCAR Surveillance Project. Semin Vasc Surg. 2020;33(1–2):24–30.
256. Ghamraoui AK, Ricotta JJ 2nd. Outcomes of Transcarotid Artery Revascularization (TCAR) in octogenarians and older. Ann Vasc Surg. 2020;68:151–8.
257. Hakimi A, Choi ES, Aziz F, Aziz F. Evolution of medical and surgical management of carotid disease—from carotid endarterectomy to transfemoral carotid stenting to TCAR. Ann Vasc Surg. 2024; https://doi.org/10.1016/j.avsg.2024.09.042.
258. Intagliata A, Rountree K, Bath J. Thrombosis or vasospasm: the utility of intraoperative neuromonitoring during TCAR. Vascular. 2023;31(4):694–8.
259. Kashyap VS, So KL, Schneider PA, Rathore R, Pham T, Motaganahalli RL, et al. One-year outcomes after Transcarotid Artery Revascularization (TCAR) in the ROADSTER 2 trial. J Vasc Surg. 2022;76(2):466–73 e1.
260. Khan MA, Elsayed N, Naazie I, Ramakrishnan G, Kashyap VS, Malas MB. Impact of frailty on postoperative outcomes in patients undergoing TransCarotid Artery Revascularization (TCAR). Ann Vasc Surg. 2022;84:126–34.
261. Naazie IN, Dodo-Williams T, Janssen C, Lane J, Smeds MR, Malas M. Impact of flow reversal duration on neurological outcomes of Transcarotid Artery Revascularization (TCAR). Ann Vasc Surg. 2023;89:11–9.
262. Oye H, Abbas N. Transcarotid Artery Revascularization (TCAR): the best surgical intervention option in an unusual presentation of carotid dissection in a 37-year-old pregnant female. Cureus. 2024;16(2):e54600.
263. Paraskevas KI, AbuRahma AF, Abularrage CJ, Clair DG, Eldrup-Jorgensen J, Kashyap VS, et al. An international, expert-based Delphi consensus document on controversial issues about TransCarotid Artery Revascularization (TCAR). Ann Vasc Surg. 2024;110:42.
264. Piper K, Farooq J, Yeung E, Flores-Milan G, Van Loveren H, Lau T. Transcarotid Artery Revascularization (TCAR) stenting or angioplasty for intracranial carotid artery stenosis: case series and novel application. Interv Neuroradiol. 2023;29(4):351–7.

265. Sato D, Umekawa M, Koizumi S, Ishigami D, Kiyofuji S, Saito N. Trans-distal radial artery carotid revascularization with forearm flow reversal: an alternative option of CAS in the TCAR era. World Neurosurg. 2024;183:e920–e7.
266. Sujijantarat N, Antonios J, Koo A, Renedo D, Cord BJ, Zetchi A, et al. Transcarotid Artery Revascularization (TCAR): a technical video. J Neurointerv Surg. 2022;14(8):842.
267. Sundaram SS, King RW, Genovese EA, Veeraswamy RK. Ultrasound examination without axial imaging is sufficient for preoperative planning in Transcarotid Artery Revascularization (TCAR). Ann Vasc Surg. 2023;97:192–202.
268. Taylor K, Mouawad NJ. Mastering Transcarotid Artery Revascularization (TCAR) instrumentation efficiency. J Vasc Nurs. 2020;38(4):180–2.
269. Teter K, Rockman C, Lamparello P, Macdonald S, Garg K, Barfield M, et al. Risk factors for and intraoperative management of intolerance to flow reversal in TCAR. Ann Vasc Surg. 2022;79:41–5.
270. Vuppala S, Kim J, Joo BS, Choi JM, Jang J. A combination of pharmacophore-based virtual screening, structure-based lead optimization, and DFT study for the identification of S. epidermidis TcaR inhibitors. Pharmaceuticals (Basel). 2022;15(5, 635)
271. Yammine H, Briggs C, Arko FR 3rd. Transcarotid Artery Revascularization (TCAR) in the frail. Ann Vasc Surg. 2022;84:135–6.
272. Loufopoulos G, Manaki V, Tasoudis P, Karela N-R, Sénéchaud C, Giannopoulos A, et al. Trans-carotid artery revascularization versus carotid endarterectomy in patients with carotid artery disease: systematic review and meta-analysis of 30-day outcomes. Angiology. 2024; https://doi.org/10.1177/00033197241241788.
273. Paraskevas KI, Malas MB, Schermerhorn ML. Transcarotid artery revascularization versus carotid endarterectomy. Angiology. 2024:33197241261453.
274. Naazie IN, Cui CL, Osaghae I, Murad MH, Schermerhorn M, Malas MB. A systematic review and meta-analysis of transcarotid artery revascularization with dynamic flow reversal versus transfemoral carotid artery stenting and carotid endarterectomy. Ann Vasc Surg. 2020;69:426–36.
275. Ghannam M, AlMajali M, Khasiyev F, Dibas M, Al Qudah A, AlMajali F, et al. Transcarotid arterial revascularization of symptomatic internal carotid artery disease: a systematic review and study-level meta-analysis. Stroke (1970). 2024;55(4):921.

Open and Endovascular Treatment of Carotid Aneurysms

8

Djordje Radak and Stevo Duvnjak

8.1 Introduction

An aneurysm is generally defined as an expansion of the arterial lumen by more than 50% of its normal diameter. However, in the case of the carotid artery, this definition varies. In the carotid artery, an aneurysm is defined as a bulbar dilation of 200% of the internal carotid artery's diameter and 150% of the common carotid artery's diameter [1]. Most aneurysms involve the bulb region and internal carotid artery, while aneurysms of the external carotid artery are very rare. Carotid aneurysm resection accounts for 0.1–3% of carotid artery surgeries [2]. The leading causes of carotid artery aneurysms include atherosclerosis, trauma, post-endarterectomy changes, congenital factors, inflammation, and fibromuscular dysplasia. Carotid artery aneurysms can be classified as either true or false [3]. True aneurysms typically develop due to atherosclerosis, arteritis, fibromuscular dysplasia, or as pseudoaneurysms. The etiology is most often post-traumatic or mycotic.

A saccular aneurysm is characterized by a segmental, lateral (asymmetric) expansion of the artery, whereas a fusiform aneurysm involves a segmental (symmetric) expansion of the artery's diameter. Fusiform aneurysms are more common than saccular ones and frequently occur at the bifurcation of the common carotid artery, while saccular aneurysms are more often found in the internal carotid artery.

D. Radak
Serbian Academy of Sciences and Arts, Belgrade, Serbia

Clinic for Surgery, Euromedik Hospital, Belgrade, Serbia
e-mail: radak@ikvbd.com

S. Duvnjak (✉)
Department of Vascular Surgery, Rigshospitalet, Copenhagen, Denmark
e-mail: stevo.duvnjak@regionh.dk

D. Radak, S. Duvnjak (eds.), *Carotid Artery Disease: Surgical Perspectives*,
https://doi.org/10.1007/978-3-031-81842-4_8

Carotid artery aneurysms can lead to severe complications, including:

- Distal embolization
- Compression symptoms
- Rupture

Most patients present with a pulsatile mass in the neck, and 12–51% may experience distal embolization and cerebral ischemia [4]. A small carotid aneurysm can be asymptomatic and discovered incidentally. Other possible symptoms may include nerve compression, dysphagia, tinnitus, hoarseness, and bleeding [5].

Small, non-growing aneurysms in asymptomatic patients may, in some cases, be managed conservatively with antiplatelet or anticoagulant medication, along with regular clinical and imaging follow-up. Color Doppler ultrasound is typically the first diagnostic modality and can effectively detect the aneurysm size, blood flow within the aneurysm, and the presence of thrombus (Fig. 8.1). Magnetic resonance imaging (MRI) and computed tomography (CT) are advanced imaging modalities that allow for detailed treatment planning and the identification of other intracranial aneurysms discovery (Fig. 8.2). Invasive angiography is typically not used solely for diagnosis today but rather as part of the treatment process.

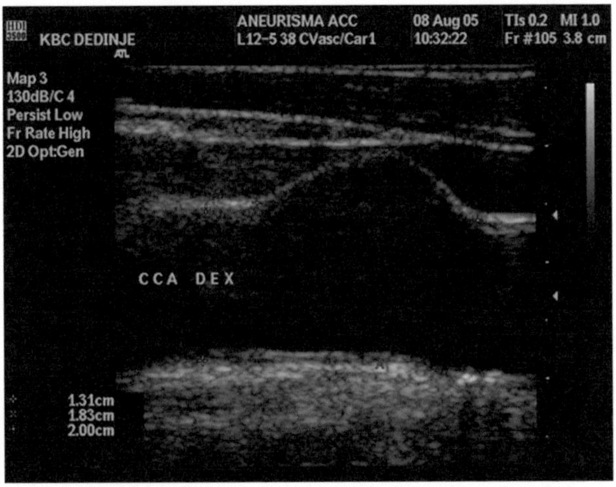

Fig. 8.1 B-mode ultrasound examination revealed a carotid artery bulb aneurysm

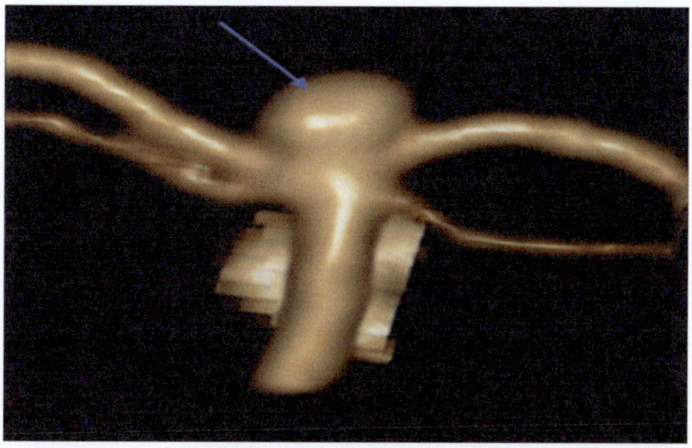

Fig. 8.2 An asymptomatic basilar artery aneurysm was incidentally discovered on a computed tomography 3D reconstruction

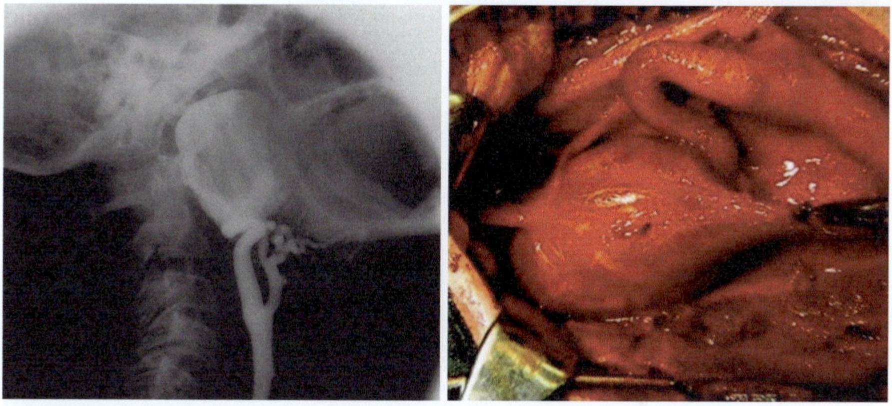

Fig. 8.3 Angiography of large distal internal carotid aneurysms and intraoperative findings

8.2 Open Surgery of Carotid Aneurysm

Surgical treatment of extracranial carotid aneurysms typically involves aneurysm resection and artery reconstruction. The treatment generally consists of aneurysm resection followed by primary repair or graft interposition. Graft materials such as Dacron, polytetrafluoroethylene (PTFE), bovine pericardium, or autologous vein can be used for carotid reconstructions. The techniques used are similar to those in endarterectomy, but aneurysm resection may require more distal exposure of the internal carotid artery, which can be challenging and necessitates careful preoperative planning.

Ligation of the carotid artery is usually reserved for cases of infection and is associated with a high complication rate (30–60%), making it a last resort when other options are not viable. The combined mortality and ischemic complication rates for carotid reconstructions can reach up to 10%, with nerve lesions occurring in up to 12% of cases [6] (Figs. 8.3 and 8.4).

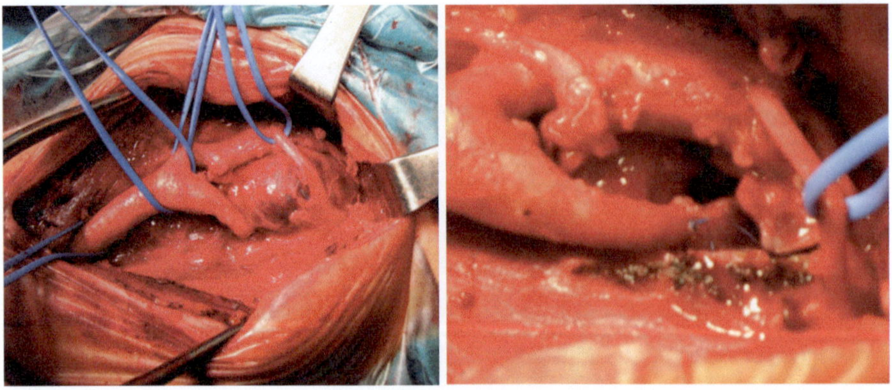

Fig. 8.4 Intraoperative views during and after carotid aneurysm resection may require extensive exposure. In some cases, “high” exposure necessitates nasotracheal intubation and division of the digastric muscle

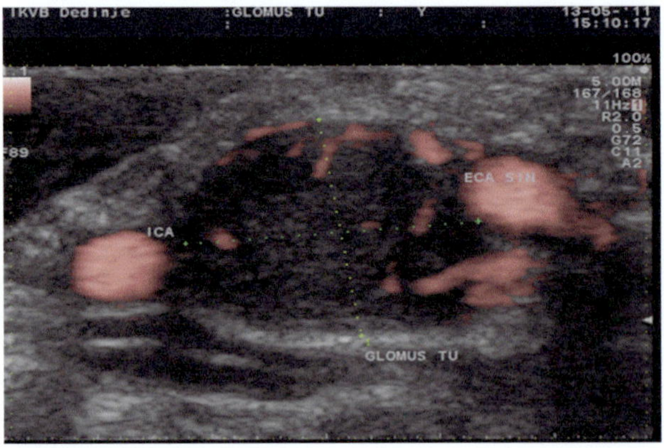

Fig. 8.5 Color Doppler ultrasound showing a hypervascular glomus tumor

Carotid body (glomus) tumors are paraganglion neoplasms originating from the cells of the carotid body. These tumors are typically located at the carotid bifurcation. They usually occur in patients aged over 40–50 years, can be bilateral in up to 10% of cases, and have a familial predisposition in approximately 25% of patients [7]. The most common clinical presentation is a slow-growing, asymptomatic, palpable, non-pulsatile mass in the neck. In larger tumors, the compression of surrounding structures such as nerves, the sympathetic chain, or the esophagus can occur. Some tumors may be hormone active and produce catecholamines. Doppler ultrasound is typically the initial diagnostic modality, as it clearly visualizes the neoplasm and allows assessment of vascularization (Fig. 8.5). Advanced imaging techniques, such as computed tomography (CT) or magnetic resonance imaging (MRI), are usually required for proper surgical planning (Fig. 8.6). In exceptional cases, positron emission tomography (PET) may be used if multiple neoplasms are suspected (Fig. 8.7). Invasive angiography is employed only if preoperative embolization is planned, not as a diagnostic procedure (Fig. 8.8). Surgery to remove the

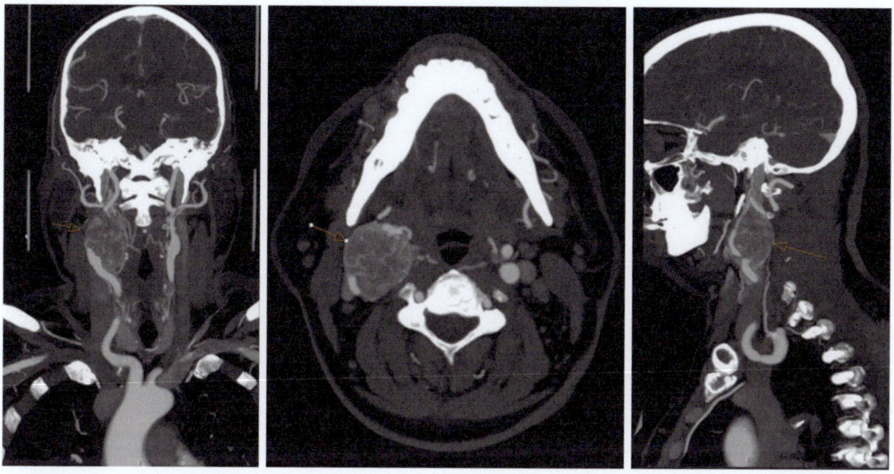

Fig. 8.6 Computed tomography in all three planes, sagittal, axial, and coronal, revealed a large Shamblin type 2 glomus tumor in close contact with the internal and external carotid arteries

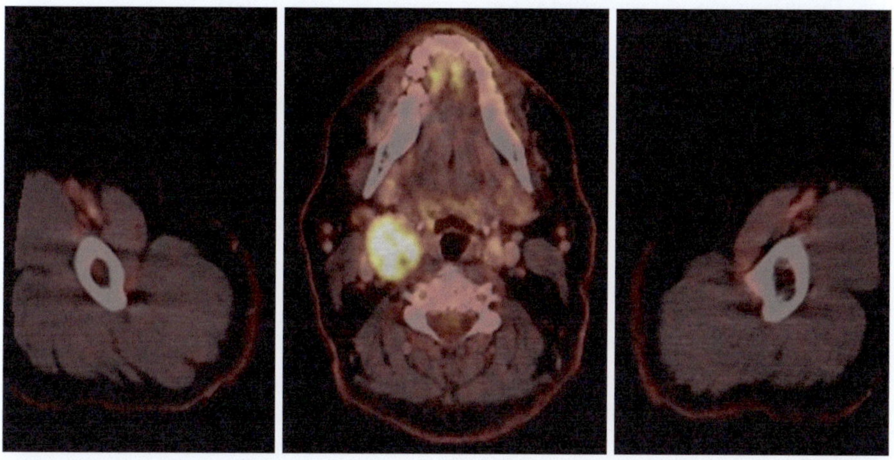

Fig. 8.7 Positron emission tomography showed increased uptake of octreoscan in the glomus tumor on the right side

tumor is the treatment of choice due to the risk of malignant transformation. The Shamblin's classification is widely used in practice, with Type I tumors being the most accessible for surgery, as they are not in close contact with the carotid artery and nerves. Shamblin types II and III are more complex and challenging to remove due to their close proximity to the carotid artery and nerves [8]. In some extreme cases of type III Shamblin tumor, ligation of the carotid artery may be the only solution. Surgery requires careful planning and usually entails higher exposure. Bleeding complications, Horner's syndrome due to sympathetic chain lesions, and nerve lesions are the most frequent issues, with nerve lesions occurring in up to 24% of

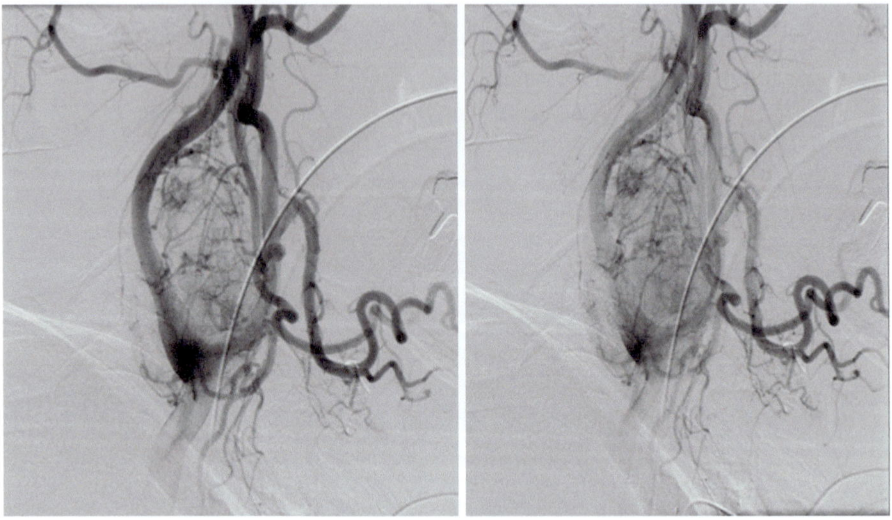

Fig. 8.8 Invasive angiography revealed a large hypervascular glomus tumor at the carotid bifurcation. The angiography was performed as part of preoperative embolization

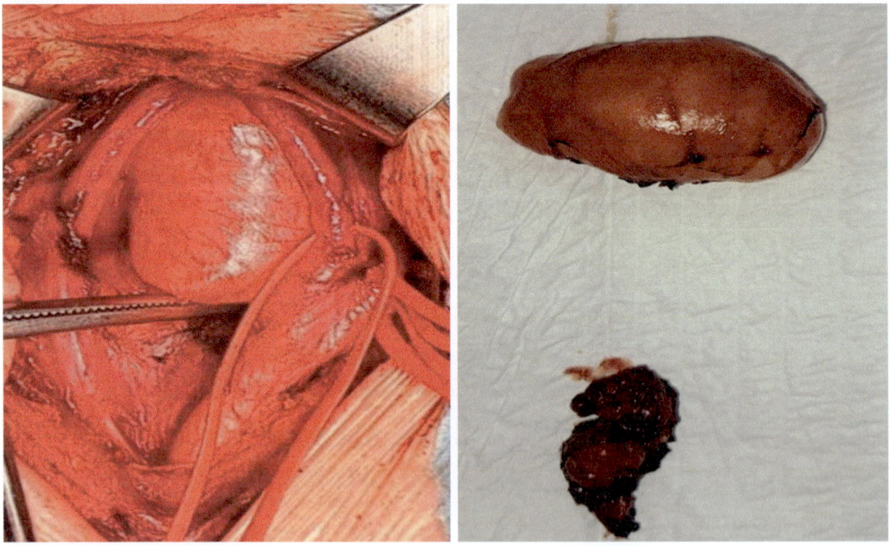

Fig. 8.9 Intraoperative findings of a non-glomus, non-malignant tumor located behind the carotid bifurcation present diagnostic challenges

cases [9]. Other specific complications include stroke in about 4% of cases and baroreceptor dysfunction in about 20% [10]. Not all neck and carotid bifurcation masses are carotid artery aneurysms or glomus tumors; other benign tumors may also be encountered during surgery (Fig. 8.9).

8.3 Endovascular Treatment of Carotid Aneurysm

Endovascular treatment is a valid option, particularly for distally located aneurysms that are inaccessible to open surgery and in cases where open surgery is considered high risk. The stent graft is the most commonly used technique, offering high technical success, though the risk of stent graft thrombosis remains a concern. Another approach is stent-assisted coil embolization and occlusion of the carotid artery. Endovascular treatment is contraindicated in cases with a large thrombus load within the aneurysm due to the risk of distal embolization and in cases of significant arterial elongation. Infective pseudoaneurysms can sometimes be definitively treated with a stent graft. Traumatic pseudoaneurysms are increasingly treated with a stent graft, provided the anatomy is suitable (Figs. 8.10 and 8.11).

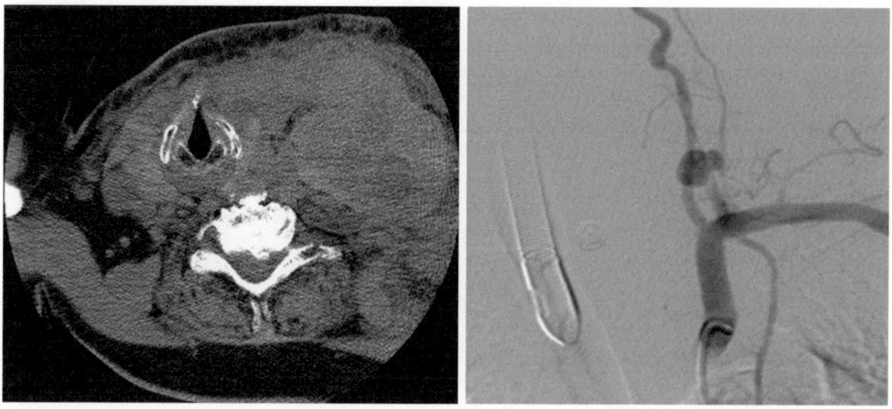

Fig. 8.10 Traumatic lesion and hematoma in the left supraclavicular region. Angiography with left vertebral artery pseudoaneurysm

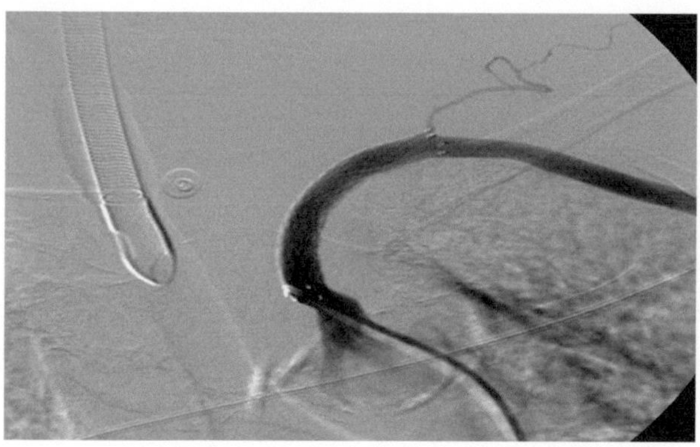

Fig. 8.11 Control after stent graft deployment and arrest bleeding

References

1. de Jong KP, Zondervan PE, van Urk H. Extracranial carotid artery aneurysms. Eur J Vasc Surg. 1989;3:557–62.
2. Welleweerd JC, den Ruijter HM, Nelissen BG, Bots ML, Kappelle LJ, Rinkel GJ, et al. Management of extracranial carotid artery aneurysm. Eur J Vasc Endovasc Surg. 2015;50:141–7.
3. Longo GM, Kibbe MR. Aneurysms of the carotid artery. Semin Vasc Surg. 2005;18:178–83.
4. Garg K, Rockman CB, Lee V, Maldonado TS, Jacobowitz GR, Adelman MA, Mussa FF. Presentation and management of carotid artery aneurysms and pseudoaneurysms. J Vasc Surg. 2012;55:1618–22.
5. Kraemer CJK, Zhou W. Carotid aneurysm review. Int J Angiol. 2019;28:17–9.
6. Welleweerd JC, den Ruijter HM, Nelissen BGL, Bots ML, Kappelle LJ, Rinkel GJE, F. L., et al. Management of extracranial carotid artery aneurysm. Eur J Vasc Endovasc Surg. 2015;2015(50):141–7.
7. Davila VJ, Chang JM, Stone WM, Fowl RJ, Bower TC, Michael L, et al. Current surgical management of carotid body tumors. J Vasc Surg. 2016;64:1703–10.
8. Shamblin WR, ReMine WH, Sheps SG, Harrison EG. Carotid body tumor (Chemodectoma). Clinicopathologic analysis of ninety cases. Am J Surg. 1971;122:732–9.
9. Kim GY, Lawrence PF, Moridzadeh RS, et al. New predictors of complications in carotid body tumor resection. J Vasc Surg. 2017;65:1673–9.
10. Cobb AN, Barkat A, Daungjaiboon W, Halandras P, Crisostomo P, Kuo PC, et al. Carotid body tumor resection: just as safe without preoperative embolisation. Ann Vasc Surg. 2017;46:54.

Treatment of Carotid Dissection

9

Djordje Radak and Stevo Duvnjak

9.1 Introduction

Spontaneous carotid dissection is a rare cause of stroke, accounting for up to 2% of cases. However, in individuals under 50 years of age, it is responsible for 25–30% of stroke symptoms [1]. Genetic factors, congenital conditions, connective tissue diseases, arterial elongation, and minor trauma are recognized as risk factors for spontaneous dissection. Carotid or vertebral dissection can lead to artery thrombosis and distal thromboembolic complications, stenosis or occlusion of the carotid/vertebral artery, and the formation of aneurysms. The mechanisms of dissection include intimal tear or vasa vasorum rupture and intramural hematoma formation, which contribute to the symptoms. Patients typically present with unilateral facial or neck pain, headache, Horner syndrome (ptosis and miosis), and nerve compression. However, dissection can also manifest as a stroke or, less commonly, as spinal ischemia [2]. Unspecified symptoms can lead to delayed diagnosis and progression of the condition. A detailed anamnesis and neurological examination are essential for diagnosing carotid dissection. Doppler ultrasound is the preferred initial diagnostic tool due to its high accuracy for carotid dissection, though it is less effective for vertebral artery dissection. Possible ultrasound findings include an intimal flap, double lumen, thrombus, stenosis/occlusion, or dissection aneurysm (see Figs. 9.1 and 9.2). Cross-sectional imaging methods, such as computed tomography (CT) and magnetic resonance angiography (MRA), are also excellent diagnostic tools.

D. Radak
Serbian Academy of Sciences and Arts, Belgrade, Serbia

Clinic for Surgery, Euromedik Hospital, Belgrade, Serbia
e-mail: radak@ikvbd.com

S. Duvnjak (✉)
Department of Vascular Surgery, Rigshospitalet, Copenhagen, Denmark
e-mail: stevo.duvnjak@regionh.dk

D. Radak, S. Duvnjak (eds.), *Carotid Artery Disease: Surgical Perspectives*,
https://doi.org/10.1007/978-3-031-81842-4_9

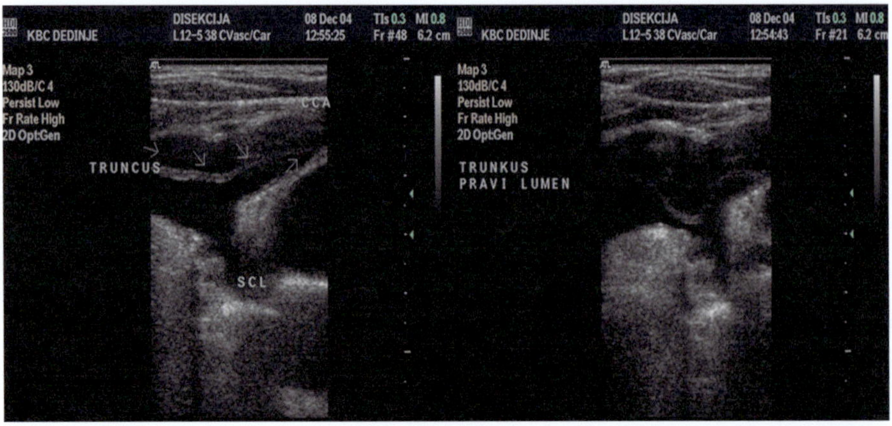

Fig. 9.1 B-mode ultrasound shows an intimal dissection flap extending from the brachiocephalic trunk into the carotid artery, with movement during the cardiac cycle

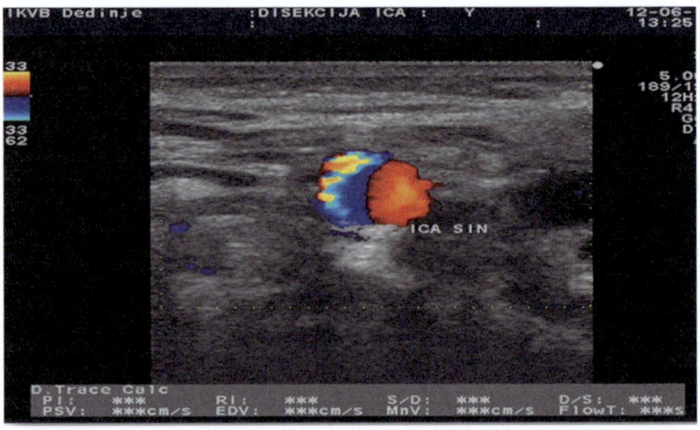

Fig. 9.2 Color Doppler shows a "double" lumen flow and an intimal flap between them

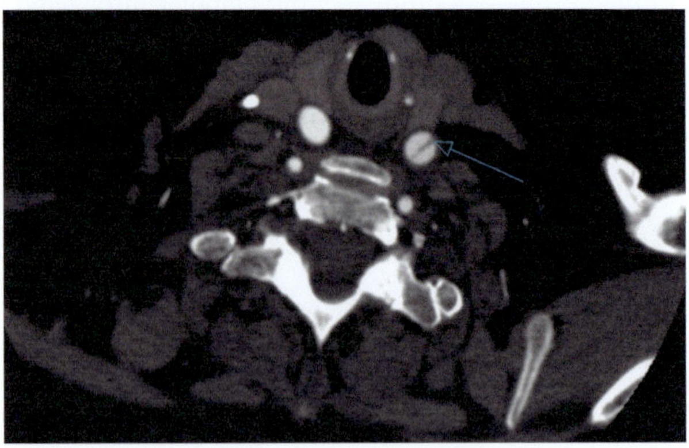

Fig. 9.3 Axial images from computed tomography show a "double" lumen indicating dissection in the left carotid artery (arrow)

CT offers the highest sensitivity and specificity for diagnosing both carotid and vertebral artery dissection (see Fig. 9.3). However, CT is less sensitive for detecting intramural hematomas, where MRA is superior. MRA, on the other hand, has lower sensitivity for vertebral artery dissection [3]. Invasive angiography is seldom used today for diagnosis and is primarily reserved for interventional procedures. Fibromuscular dysplasia of the carotid artery is a noninflammatory, nonatherosclerotic condition that primarily affects women and can be complicated by spontaneous carotid dissection in about 10% of cases.

The majority of patients with carotid or vertebral dissection experience ischemic stroke within the first 2 weeks after the onset of symptoms. Therefore, it is crucial to establish a rapid diagnosis and initiate antithrombotic therapy. However, the time interval for starting treatment can range from a few minutes to 31 days [4].

Imaging features associated with high risk include multiple dissections, vertebral artery dissection, intraluminal thrombus, and severe stenosis. These features can be used to predict the risk of developing an ischemic stroke [5].

Treatment options for carotid and vertebral dissection include:

- Conservative
- Endovascular
- Open surgical

9.2 Conservative Treatment of Carotid Dissection

Antithrombotic therapy is indicated for secondary stroke prevention in patients with carotid and vertebral artery dissection. Both antiplatelet and anticoagulant medications can be used. Data from two randomized studies, the Cervical Artery Dissection in Stroke Study (CADISS) and Biomarkers and Antithrombotic Treatment in Cervical Artery Dissection (TREAT-CAD), have shown no significant difference in ipsilateral stroke prevention, major intracerebral bleeding, or mortality between anticoagulant and antiplatelet treatments [6, 7].

If anticoagulant medication is used, the International Normalized Ratio (INR) should be maintained at 2.5 (with a range of 2–3). For antiplatelet therapy, aspirin is typically administered at 75–300 mg and clopidogrel at 75 mg.

Dual antiplatelet therapy with aspirin and clopidogrel can be prescribed for 30–90 days if there are no bleeding risks, after which monotherapy is generally recommended. The optimal duration of antiplatelet therapy remains debated, but it is typically administered for at least 3–6 months, or as a permanent monotherapy based on an individualized approach.

Ultrasound control is usually performed 3 or 6 months later, as most dissections stabilize within this timeframe. The risk of recurrent dissection is approximately 3.3%, often with a benign course. Predictors of recurrent dissection include fibromuscular dysplasia, younger age, and migraine [8].

There is no randomized comparison between vitamin K antagonists and non-vitamin K oral anticoagulants (NOACs). However, published data indicate a slightly higher risk of extracranial bleeding with vitamin K antagonists, while there is no significant difference in stroke prevention between the two groups [9].

Traumatic carotid dissection is a distinct condition, but its clinical presentation and treatment are similar to those of spontaneous dissection.

9.3 Operative Treatment of Carotid Dissection

Operative treatment of carotid dissection is indicated only if symptoms persist or recur after initiating medical antithrombotic therapy. Dissection aneurysms rarely expand or cause pressure symptoms, and rupture is uncommon. If the patient has contraindications to antithrombotic therapy, those with ischemic stroke complications who are candidates for thrombolysis or mechanical thrombectomy in acute settings should undergo endovascular treatment, including thrombectomy and stent placement (Figs. 9.4, 9.5, and 9.6).

In subacute cases, if symptoms persist or recur, an endovascular stent may be deployed in selected patients. Open-operative surgery, which includes endarterectomy with patch angioplasty, carotid artery bypass, aneurysm resection, or carotid artery ligation if feasible, is now rare for carotid dissection cases.

Traumatic or iatrogenic carotid dissection can lead to severe complications and outcomes despite treatment (see Figs. 9.7 and 9.8).

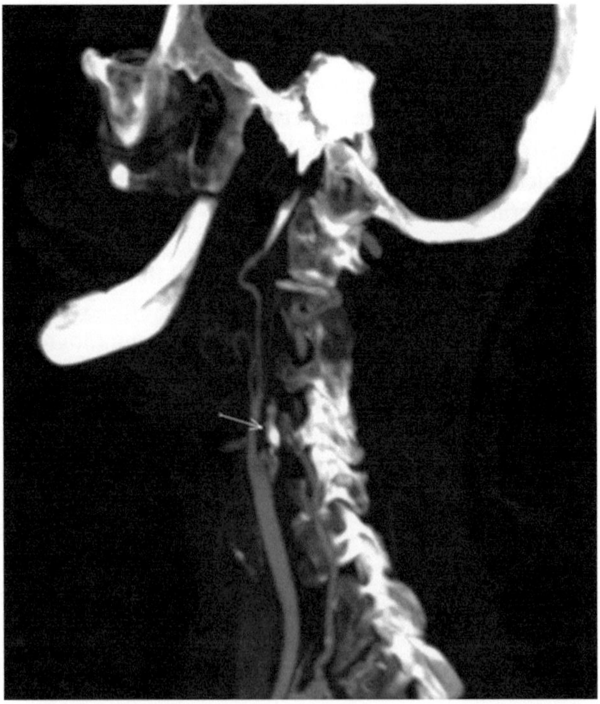

Fig. 9.4 Acute internal carotid dissection with complete occlusion of the internal carotid artery, leading to an ischemic stroke. The white arrow indicates the site of occlusion in the internal carotid artery

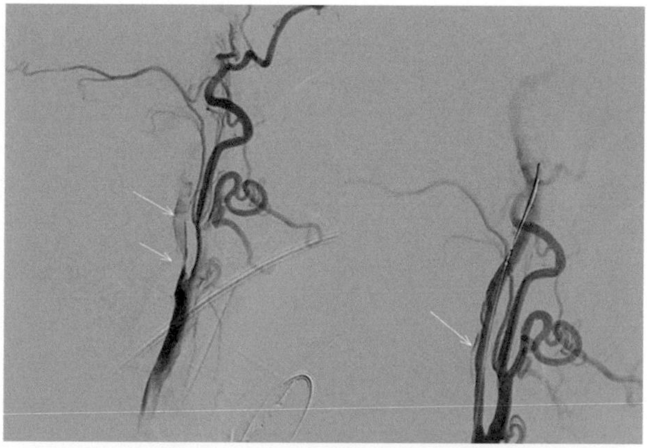

Fig. 9.5 Angiography shows carotid dissection and intraluminal thrombus (indicated by white arrows)

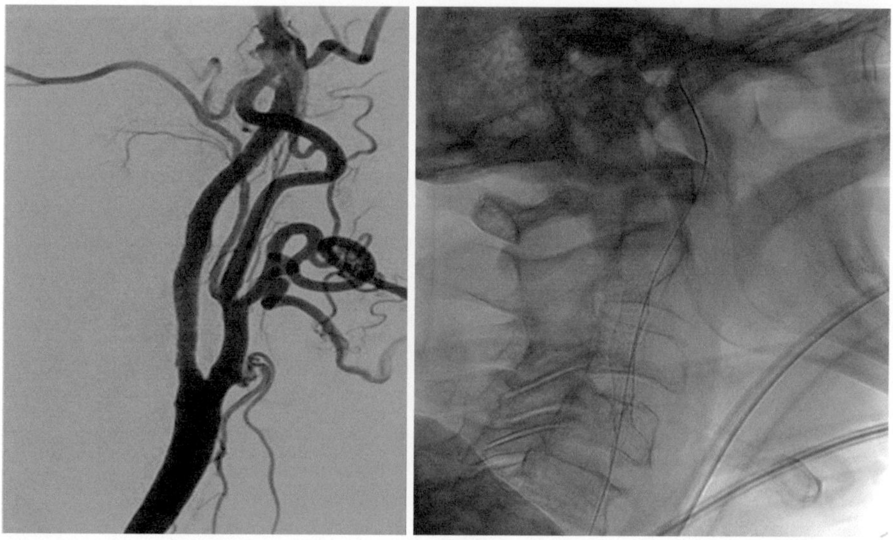

Fig. 9.6 Control angiography after stent deployment shows restoration of lumen and flow in the internal carotid artery

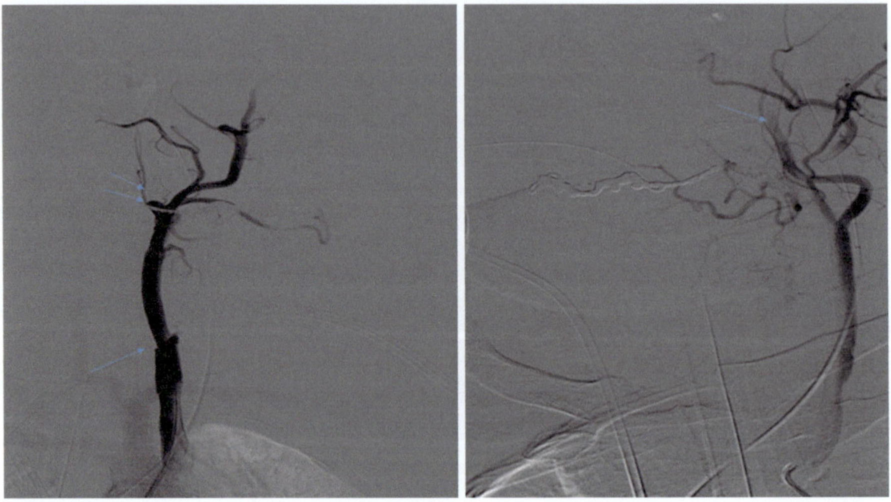

Fig. 9.7 Iatrogenic dissection of the common and internal carotid arteries with occlusion of the internal carotid artery and thrombus formation (indicated by arrows)

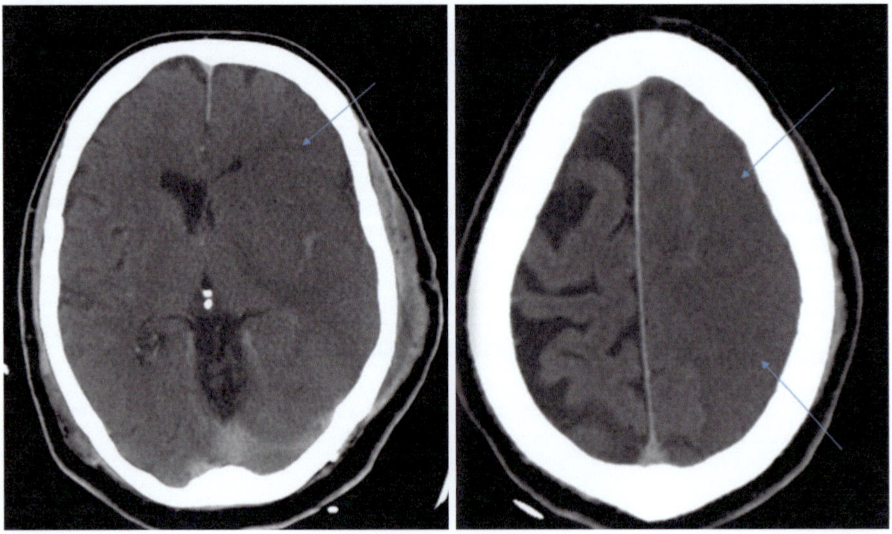

Fig. 9.8 Despite the stent deployment, a massive infarct occurred in the left cerebral hemisphere

References

1. Ekker MS, Verhoeven JI, Schellekens MMI, Boot EM, van Alebeek ME, Brouwers PJAM, et al. Risk factors and causes of ischemic stroke in 1322 young adults. Stroke. 2023;54:439–47.
2. Mokri B, Silbert PL, Schievink WI, Piepgras DG. Cranial nerve palsy in spontaneous dissection of the extracranial internal carotid artery. Neurology. 1996;46:366–59.
3. Chen CJ, Tseng YC, Lee TH, Hsu HL, See LC. Multisection CT angiography compared with catheter angiography in diagnosis vertebral artery dissection. Am J Neuroradiol. 2004;25:769–74.
4. Biousse V, Anglejan-Chatilon DJ, Touboul PJ, Amarenco P, Bousser MG. Time course of symptoms in extracranial carotid artery dissection: a series of 80 patients. Stroke. 1995;26:235–9.
5. Yaghi S, Engelter S, Del Brutto VJ, Field TS, Jadhav AP, Kicielinski K, American Heart Association Stroke Council; Council on Cardiovascular and Stroke Nursing; Council on Clinical Cardiology; and Council on Peripheral Vascular Disease, et al. Treatment and outcomes of cervical artery dissection in adults: a scientific statement from the American Heart Association. Stroke. 2024;55:e91–e106.
6. CADISS Trial Investigators, et al. Antiplatelet treatment compared with anticoagulation treatment for cervical artery dissection (CADISS): a randomised trial. Lancet Neurol. 2015;14(4):361–7.
7. Debette S, Mazighi M, Bijlenga P, Pezzini A, Koga M, Bersano A, et al. ESO guideline for the management of extracranial and intracranial artery dissection. Eur Stroke J. 2021;6:XXXIX–LXXXVII.
8. Huart J, Stoenoiu MS, Zedde M, Pascarella R, Adlam D, Persu A. From fibromuscular dysplasia to arterial dissection and back. Am J Hypertens. 2023;36:573–85.
9. Caprio FZ, Bernstein RA, Alberts MJ, Curran Y, Bergman D, Korutz AW, et al. Efficacy and safety of novel oral anticoagulants in patients with cervical artery dissections. Cerebrovasc Dis. 2014;38:247–53.

Vasculitis Treatment

10

Djordje Radak and Stevo Duvnjak

10.1 Introduction

Vasculitis is a noninfective systemic disease characterized by inflammation of vessels of various diameters. It can be idiopathic or secondary to other systemic diseases. Two types of vasculitis that typically involve the supra-aortic vessels are giant cell arteritis and Takayasu's arteritis. The Chapel Hill Consensus Conference on the Nomenclature of Vasculitides has effectively classified different types of vasculitis based on vessel diameter and localization [1].

Giant cell arteritis and Takayasu's arteritis are both granulomatous inflammations of the aorta and its major branches, sharing complex pathophysiology, similar clinical presentations, imaging features, and treatments. However, there are some differences: giant cell arteritis typically occurs in patients over 50 years old, with a female predominance, while Takayasu's arteritis is more common in a younger, primarily female population aged 15–30 years, particularly of Asian origin [2]. The common symptoms of giant cell arteritis include headache, jaw pain, and scalp tenderness, with elevated C-reactive protein levels in 95% of cases. Additionally, approximately 15% of patients experience ischemic ophthalmologic complications, which can lead to partial or complete visual loss [3]. Giant cell arteritis can lead to transient ischemic attacks or strokes in 2–7% of patients, either due to direct endothelial damage or a hypercoagulable state. Aortic aneurysm and dissection complications can occur in up to 30% of cases [4].

D. Radak
Serbian Academy of Sciences and Arts, Belgrade, Serbia

Clinic for Surgery, Euromedik Hospital, Belgrade, Serbia
e-mail: radak@ikvbd.com

S. Duvnjak (✉)
Department of Vascular Surgery, Rigshospitalet, Copenhagen, Denmark
e-mail: stevo.duvnjak@regionh.dk

D. Radak, S. Duvnjak (eds.), *Carotid Artery Disease: Surgical Perspectives*,
https://doi.org/10.1007/978-3-031-81842-4_10

Takayasu's arteritis typically presents with nonspecific inflammatory symptoms such as myalgia or other systemic manifestations. Symptoms of Takayasu's arteritis may include headache, syncope, convulsions, and visual disturbances. Transient ischemic attacks or strokes occur in 10–20% of patients with Takayasu's arteritis. Additionally, stenotic lesions in medium to large vessels are commonly observed in these patients [5]. Doppler ultrasound examination (Fig. 10.1), computed tomography (CT) (Fig. 10.2), magnetic resonance imaging (MRI), and positron emission tomography (PET-CT) (Fig. 10.3) play a role in diagnosing various types of vasculitis, as well as in monitoring and assessing treatment. Stenosis, aneurysm development in large vessels, wall thickening, and contrast enhancement can be observed on CT/MRI imaging.

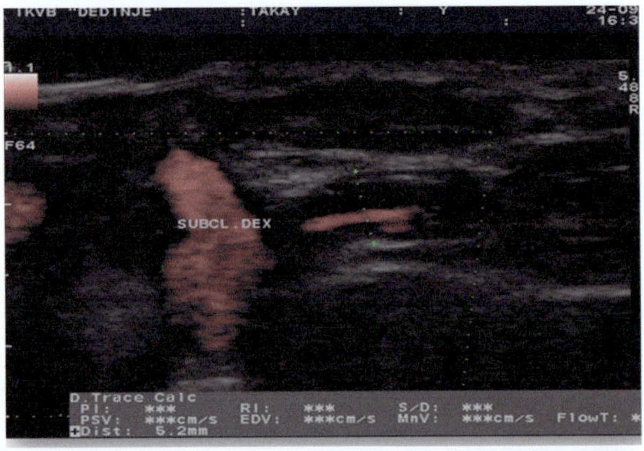

Fig. 10.1 Doppler ultrasound with wall thickening and significant stenosis of the right subclavian artery in a patient with Takayasu's arteritis

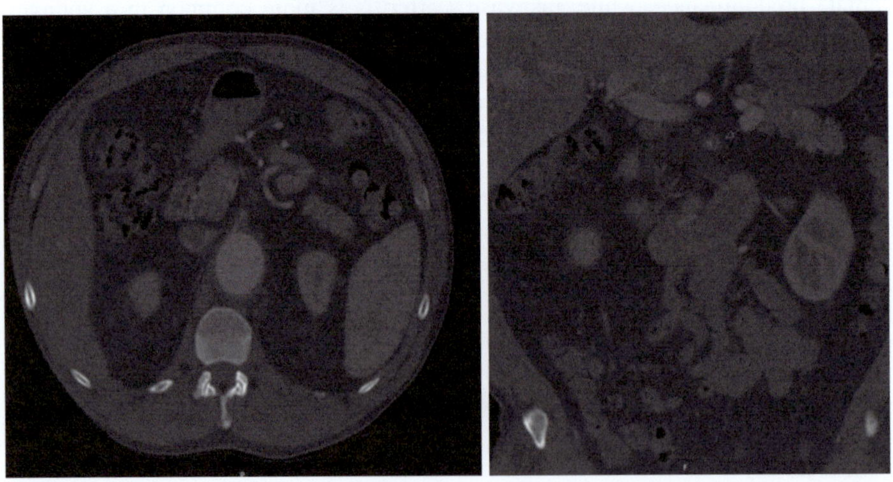

Fig. 10.2 Axial and coronal CT reconstructions show segmental stenosis and wall thickening of the superior mesenteric artery in a patient with vasculitis

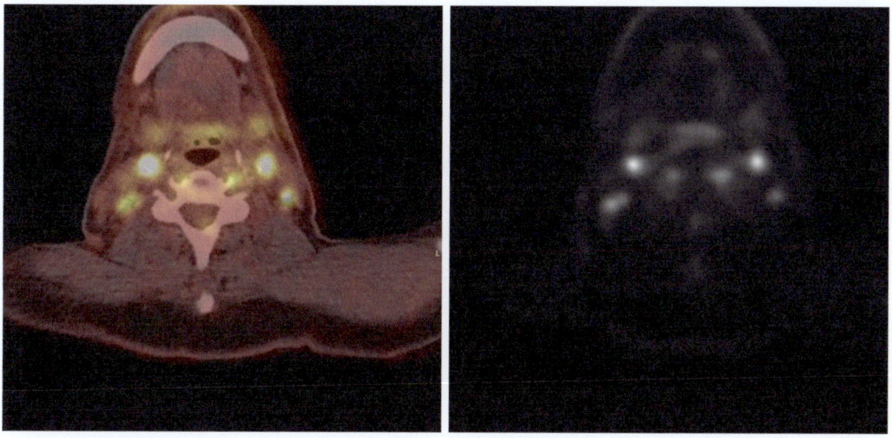

Fig. 10.3 A PET-CT scan in the acute phase of vasculitis shows increased fluorodeoxyglucose (18F-FDG) uptake in the carotid and vertebral arteries

10.2 Conservative Treatment of Vasculitis

Steroid medication is a cornerstone of vasculitis treatment. In the acute phase, high doses of prednisolone, typically 40–60 mg, are recommended. For patients with ischemic visual symptoms, a dose of 1 mg/kg of prednisolone is usually recommended for 3 days. Following this, the dose is gradually reduced to 15–20 mg for 2–3 months and then further tapered down to 5 mg [6]. Other immunosuppressive drugs used in the treatment of vasculitis include methotrexate and tocilizumab. While antiplatelet medications are prescribed for these patients, there is no strong evidence supporting their use in vasculitis.

10.3 Operative Treatment of Carotid Vasculitis

Open surgical treatment for patients with vasculitis is reserved only for severe symptomatic cases that are resistant to medical therapy and should be avoided if symptoms permit. Surgical treatment typically involves bypass procedures using usually autologous vein material. Endovascular treatment, including balloon dilation with or without a stent, can occasionally be used for patients with giant cell arteritis. However, the results for patients with Takayasu's arteritis treated endovascularly are generally unsatisfactory, and endovascular treatment is not recommended for this condition [3].

References

1. Jennette JC, Falk RJ, Bacon PA, Basu N, Cid MC, Ferrario F, et al. 2012 revised International Chapel Hill Consensus Conference Nomenclature of Vasculitides. Arthritis Rheum. 2013;65:1–11.

2. Stamatis P. Giant cell arteritis versus Takayasu arteritis: an update. Mediterr J Rheumatol. 2020;31:174–82.
3. Saadoun D, Vautier M, Cacoub P. Medium- and large-vessel vasculitis. Circulation. 2021;143(3):267–82.
4. Rüegg S, Engelter S, Jeanneret C, Hetzel A, Probst A, Steck AJ, Lyrer P. Bilateral vertebral artery occlusion resulting from giant cell arteritis: report of 3 cases and review of the literature. Medicine (Baltimore). 2003;82:1–12.
5. Duarte MM, Geraldes R, Sousa R, Alarcão J, Costa J. Stroke and transient ischemic attack in Takayasu's arteritis: a systematic review and meta-analysis. J Stroke Cerebrovasc Dis. 2016;25:781–91.
6. Hellmich B, Aqueda A, Monti S, Buttgereit F, de Boysson H, Brouwer E, et al. 2018 update of the EULAR recommendations for managing large vessel vasculitis. Ann Rheum Dis. 2020;79:19–30.

11 Subclavian and Vertebral Artery Stenosis

Djordje Radak and Stevo Duvnjak

11.1 Introduction

The supra-aortic branches are large arterial vessels originating from the aortic arch that supply blood to the head and upper extremities. These branches include the **brachiocephalic trunk**, the **left common carotid artery**, and the **left subclavian artery**. In a broader context, the **vertebral arteries** are also considered part of the supra-aortic branches.

There are notable anatomical variations in these arteries. One common variation is the **bovine arch**, where the left common carotid artery either shares a common trunk with the brachiocephalic artery or arises directly from the brachiocephalic artery. This variation is observed in up to 20% of the population [1]. Furthermore, the left vertebral artery can arise directly from the aortic arch in up to 6% of individuals, while the right subclavian artery may arise as the last branch from the aortic arch, a condition known as an aberrant right subclavian artery or arteria lusoria, occurring in about 0.6% of the population [2]. Atherosclerotic lesions in these large arteries are most common at their proximal segments, where they branch off from the aorta. Such lesions are more frequent in the left subclavian artery and the brachiocephalic trunk due to turbulence in the arterial flow at these bifurcation points. Occlusive atherosclerotic disease of the supra-aortic branches is significantly less common than carotid bifurcation lesions, occurring in 0.5–6.4% of cases, and can involve single or multiple vessels [3]. Other diseases affecting the supra-aortic branches, such as

D. Radak
Serbian Academy of Sciences and Arts, Belgrade, Serbia

Clinic for Surgery, Euromedik Hospital, Belgrade, Serbia
e-mail: radak@ikvbd.com

S. Duvnjak (✉)
Department of Vascular Surgery, Rigshospitalet, Copenhagen, Denmark
e-mail: stevo.duvnjak@regionh.dk

D. Radak, S. Duvnjak (eds.), *Carotid Artery Disease: Surgical Perspectives*, https://doi.org/10.1007/978-3-031-81842-4_11

aneurysms, dissections, compressive syndromes of the upper thoracic cavity, and various types of vasculitis, are less common. Fortunately, most lesions are segmental, which offers opportunities for intervention in symptomatic patients.

11.2 Symptoms and Indications for the Treatment

A thorough clinical examination provides crucial information about the supra-aortic arteries supplying the brain and upper extremities. The assessment should include:

- **Palpation** of the subclavian, axillary, brachial, and radial arteries in both arms to evaluate pulse quality.
- **Auscultation** of the subclavian arteries to detect any systolic murmurs.
- **Bilateral measurement** of arterial pressure, as a significant drop (more than 10–15 mmHg) in pressure in one arm compared to the other may indicate substantial narrowing of the subclavian artery. Such a drop is often associated with symptoms like fainting and dizziness.

Additionally, **clinical tests** such as the hyperabduction test and Adson's test can help identify compression in the upper thoracic outlet area [4].

The carotid system connects with the vertebrobasilar arteries at the base of the brain, forming the Circle of Willis, an irregular polygon-shaped arterial circle. This vital network facilitates the redistribution of arterial blood through the anterior, middle, and posterior cerebral arteries. Such communication allows for compensation for blockages or issues in one artery by redirecting blood flow from other arteries.

The **anterior segment** of the Circle of Willis includes the terminal branches of the right and left internal carotid arteries, the initial segments of both anterior cerebral arteries, and the anterior communicating artery, which connects the two anterior cerebral arteries. The **posterior segment** is composed of the right and left posterior communicating arteries and the basilar artery [5].

The **carotid basin** supplies the cerebrum's hemispheres, midbrain, basal ganglia, eyes, and face, so symptoms arising from this area typically reflect issues in these centers. Thromboembolic complications in the carotid basin usually present as transient ischemic attacks (TIAs) or strokes, leading to motor or sensory deficits in the extremities, as well as visual and speech difficulties.

In contrast, the **vertebrobasilar basin** nourishes the brainstem, cerebellum, medulla oblongata, and occipital lobes. Consequently, symptoms of vertebrobasilar insufficiency include dizziness, transient visual disturbances (such as flashes, scotomas, complete loss of vision, or hemianopsia), ataxia, syncope (due to disruption of the syncopal reflex in the brainstem), drop attacks (sudden falls without loss of consciousness), diplopia, dysarthria, cranial nerve dysfunction, instability while walking, contralateral or bilateral hemiparesis or hemihypesthesia, transient global amnesia, and occipital headaches.

Vascular dementia can also present suddenly and progress gradually, with acute onset followed by stepwise decline in cognitive functions, emotional instability, and relatively preserved essential personality traits.

Global Brain Ischemia arises from a general reduction in cerebral blood flow due to multi-vessel arterial stenoses or occlusions. The extent of ischemic brain lesions, as well as the type and duration of symptoms, is influenced by several factors including the severity and length of the stenosis, the effectiveness of the collateral circulation, and systemic blood pressure.

Subclavian Steal Syndrome is caused by occlusion of the proximal part of the subclavian artery, leading to "blood theft" from the cerebral circulation to the upper extremity, provided the cerebral circulation remains preserved at the level of the Willis circle. On physical examination, a weakened radial pulse may be palpable on the side of the subclavian artery stenosis, and it may be absent if the subclavian artery is occluded. Blood pressure should be measured in both arms, as it tends to be lower on the side of the occlusion.

Redirection of blood from the brain to the upper limb's vascular system can result in symptoms of cerebral ischemia, such as dizziness, fainting, and syncope. Symptoms may include both vertebrobasilar ischemia and ischemia in the ipsilateral arm.

Asymptomatic Subclavian Steal Syndrome involves occlusion of the proximal subclavian artery with retrograde flow through the ipsilateral vertebral artery, but without subjective complaints. Functional tests, such as elevation of the extremities, muscle activation, and rapid opening and closing of the hand, can reveal symptoms. These tests increase the demand for blood in the upper extremities, leading to greater "stolen" arterial blood from the intracranial circulation through the basilar and vertebral arteries, potentially provoking transient neurological symptoms. Additionally, upper extremity ischemia may manifest as activity-related fatigue, distal thromboembolic complications, or coronary ischemia in patients with an internal mammary artery bypass graft.

11.2.1 Indications for Treatment

- **Symptomatic Patients**: Those with supra-aortic vessel stenosis and focal or global neurological deficits, upper extremity ischemia, or arm fatigue, or those experiencing embolic complications.
- **Patients with Internal Mammary Artery Bypass**: Those requiring intervention to ensure good inflow if the subclavian artery is stenosed.
- **Asymptomatic Patients**: Typically managed conservatively.

11.3 Diagnosis and Treatment

Doppler ultrasound is typically the first diagnostic modality used in symptomatic patients following clinical examination (see Figs. 11.1 and 11.2). It can identify supra-aortic vessel stenosis through high peak velocity in some cases (see Fig. 11.3). More commonly, it indirectly indicates proximal stenosis or occlusion by showing a monophasic or biphasic waveform and reduced flow signal in the distal carotid,

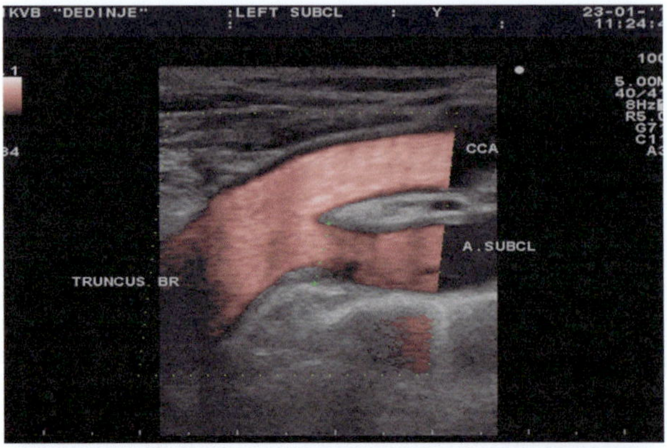

Fig. 11.1 Power Doppler examination of the brachiocephalic trunk, proximal right common carotid artery and right subclavian artery without significant stenosis

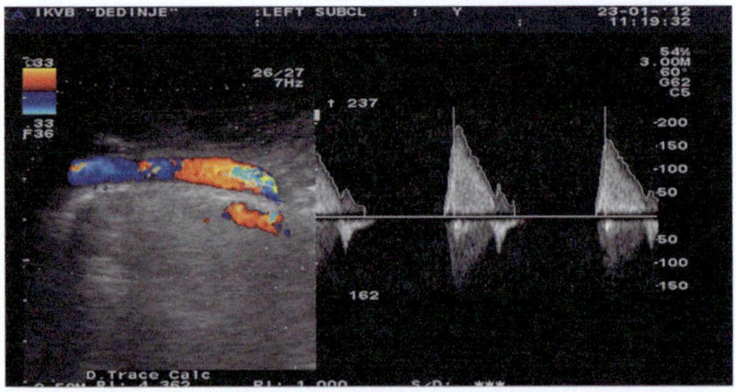

Fig. 11.2 Color Doppler analysis of the left subclavian artery showed no significant stenosis and a triphasic wave form

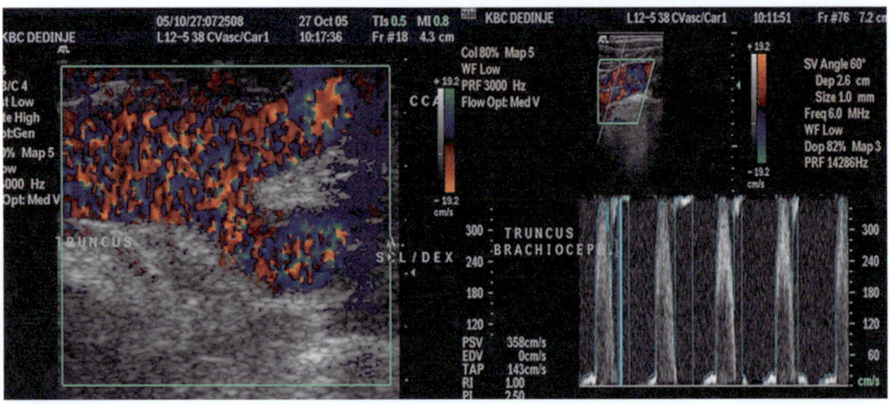

Fig. 11.3 Color Doppler and spectral analysis revealed significant stenosis (>70%) of the brachiocephalic trunk

subclavian, axillary, brachial, or radial arteries (see Fig. 11.4). Additionally, reverse flow through the vertebral artery, characteristic of subclavian steal syndrome, is effectively diagnosed using ultrasound.

Cross-sectional imaging techniques, including computed tomography (CT) and magnetic resonance angiography (MRI), are essential for diagnosis and treatment planning. CT is particularly valuable and more frequently utilized. It provides detailed information on single or multi-vessel disease, ulcerated plaques, the length of stenosis or occlusion, the status of the Willis circle, aortic arch calcification, and the origin of supra-aortic branches (see Figs. 11.5 and 11.6).

Invasive angiography is integral to the treatment process and is not used solely for diagnosis. Additionally, CT scans are useful for follow-up control and for diagnosing significant stent stenosis (Fig. 11.7).

Surgical treatment for symptomatic supra-aortic vessel diseases involves several approaches: intrathoracic ascending aorta exposure, bypass surgery to the supra-aortic vessels, and cervical approaches, including various bypass operations and vessel transposition.

Intrathoracic Exposure: This approach is typically used for multi-level or severely calcified supra-aortic disease and usually requires a transsternal thoracotomy with proximal anastomosis to the ascending aorta. While this technique is a significant operation with excellent long-term results, it carries increased morbidity. It can be combined with thoracic endovascular stent deployment when there is an insufficient proximal landing zone in conjunction with supra-aortic vessel transposition surgery (Fig. 11.8).

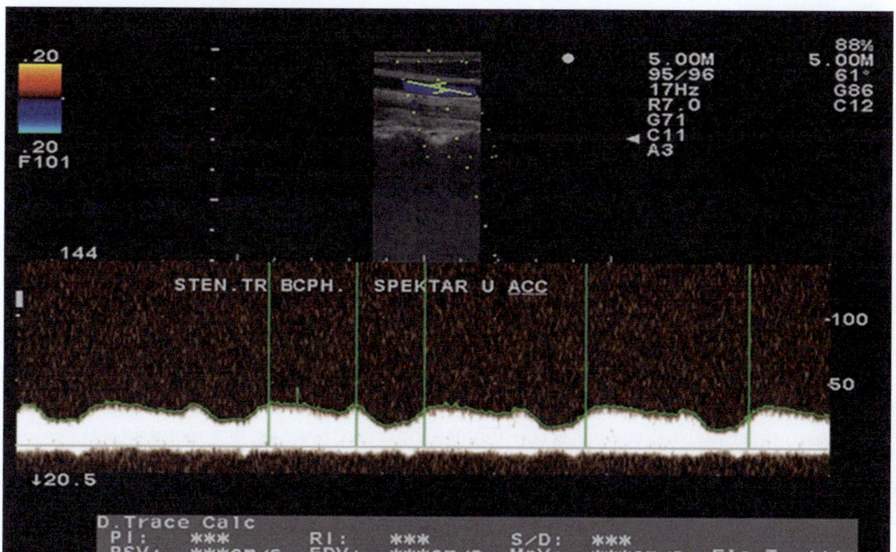

Fig. 11.4 Indirect indicator for significant proximal stenosis of the brachiocephalic trunk. Spectral analysis of the right common carotid artery, performed distally, shows a monophasic spectrum, which suggests significant proximal stenosis of the brachiocephalic trunk

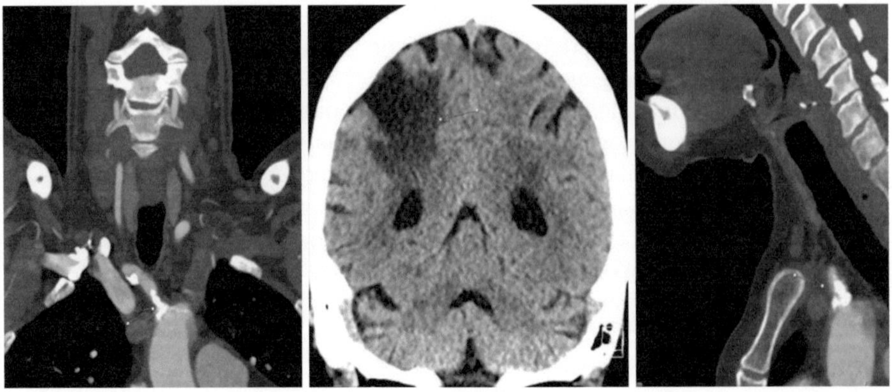

Fig. 11.5 Significant stenosis of the brachiocephalic trunk, complicated by dense calcifications, has led to an ischemic stroke in the right hemisphere. This lesion is unsuitable for surgical endarterectomy and would be better addressed with transthoracic exposure and bypass from the ascending aorta to the carotid artery. Endovascular treatment remains an option but carries an increased risk of embolic complications. Alternatively, a hybrid approach could be considered, involving surgical exposure of the common carotid artery combined with stent deployment through the carotid artery. However, this approach also poses a risk of embolic complications in the vertebral arteries

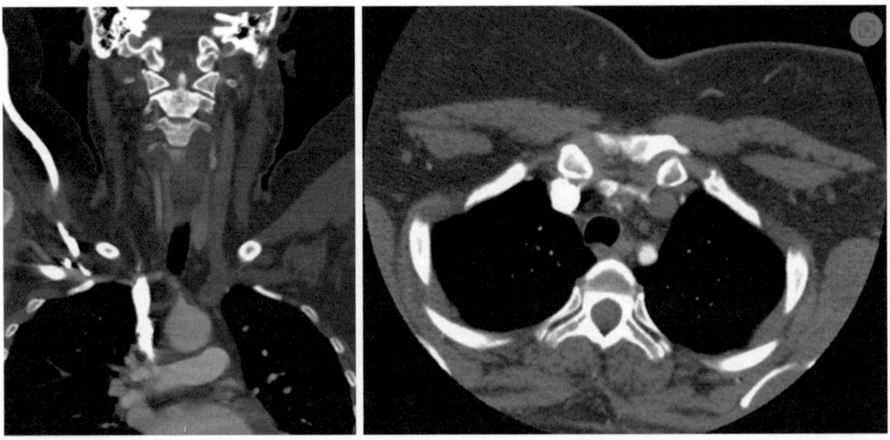

Fig. 11.6 Significant focal stenosis of the brachiocephalic trunk without associated calcification has led to ischemia in the right upper extremity. Endovascular stent deployment is indicated and can be performed via percutaneous access through the radial, brachial, or femoral artery

Cervical Approach: This option is suitable for single-vessel diseases and includes procedures such as carotid-subclavian, carotid-carotid, or axillary bypasses. Although these procedures may have slightly reduced patency compared to intrathoracic reconstructions, they involve less surgical trauma.

In the upper thoracic outlet, where four large arteries are closely positioned, the stenotic segment of one artery can sometimes be bridged by anastomosing it with an

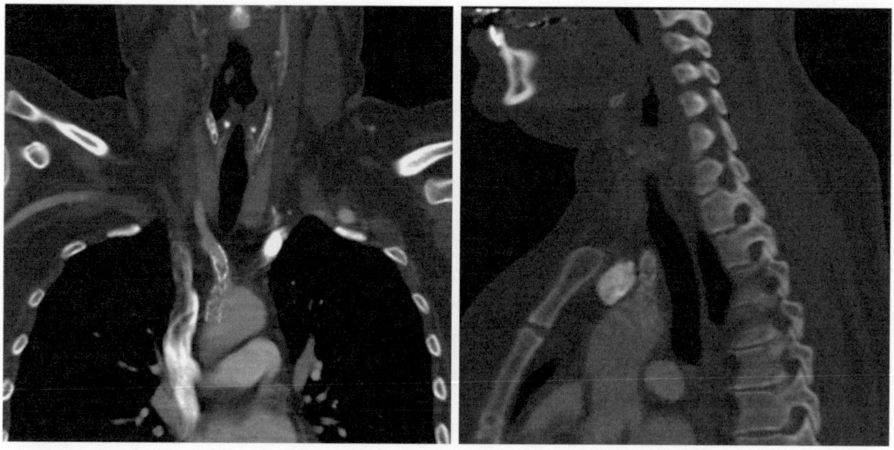

Fig. 11.7 The follow-up computed tomography scan revealed significant in-stent stenosis in the brachiocephalic trunk and recurring ischemia in the upper extremity. The stent is noted to be excessively long, protruding into the aortic lumen. Ideally, stent protrusion into the aorta should be limited to only a few millimeters. The recommended treatment involves repeat endovascular procedures, either balloon angioplasty or deployment of a new stent

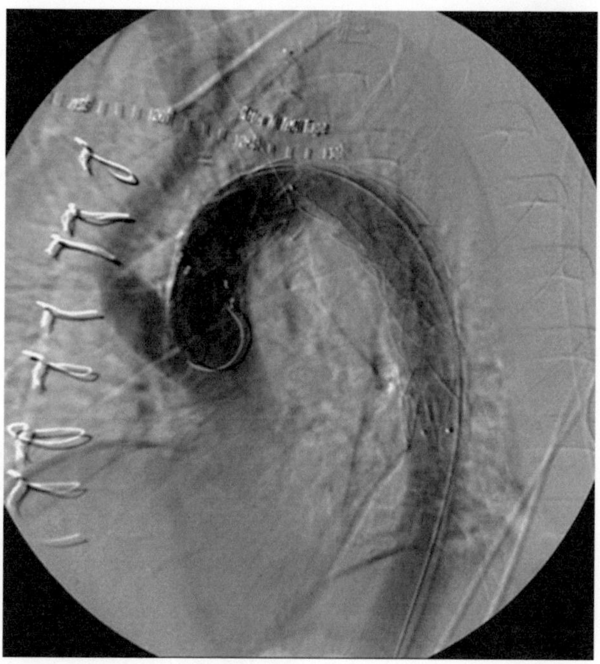

Fig. 11.8 Complete transposition of the supra-aortic vessels and afterwards TEVAR stent graft deployment

adjacent, unchanged artery. This approach allows for various elegant and creative surgical solutions. Importantly, vessel transposition does not require chest opening or thoracotomy.

By performing a transposition without a bypass graft, the operative trauma is minimal, thus avoiding the use of a foreign body. Additionally, the early and long-term results are generally better compared to transthoracic and extra-anatomical reconstructions.

Left subclavian or vertebral artery transposition is an example of such surgery, which generally yields good results. However, anatomical restrictions may make this procedure unsuitable for every patient (Fig. 11.9).

Bypass reconstruction of diseased or injured arterial segments in the supra-aortic trunks requires significant surgical skill and precision. Synthetic grafts are used to bridge the arterial segments of the larger supra-aortic branches up to the level of the carotid bifurcation. These arteries have high flow rates, and the long-term outcomes with synthetic grafts are generally superior to those of peripheral arterial reconstructions. Synthetic grafts are less susceptible to dilation, rupture, kinking, and external compression compared to autogenous grafts.

Bypass operations on supra-aortic branches can be performed through transthoracic approaches (requiring sternotomy or thoracotomy) or transcervical approaches (accessing the arteries through the neck).

Endovascular treatment for symptomatic supra-aortic vessel diseases typically involves angioplasty with primary stent deployment, which yields better results than balloon angioplasty alone. Currently, endovascular treatment is often the preferred option if the characteristics of the lesion permit.

A balloon-expandable stent is typically used for ostial lesions, while a self-expandable stent is preferred for longer lesions. Stent grafts are an effective option for high-embolic-risk ulcerated plaques. Although drug-eluting stents and balloons are available, they are rarely used in supra-aortic vessels. Treatment is performed via transfemoral (Fig. 11.10) or transradial/brachial access (Fig. 11.11), with balloons and stents available in sizes such as 0.035, 0.014, or 0.018 in.

Preoperative computed tomography scan analysis is essential for planning and executing interventions with minimal risk and complications. Thromboembolic

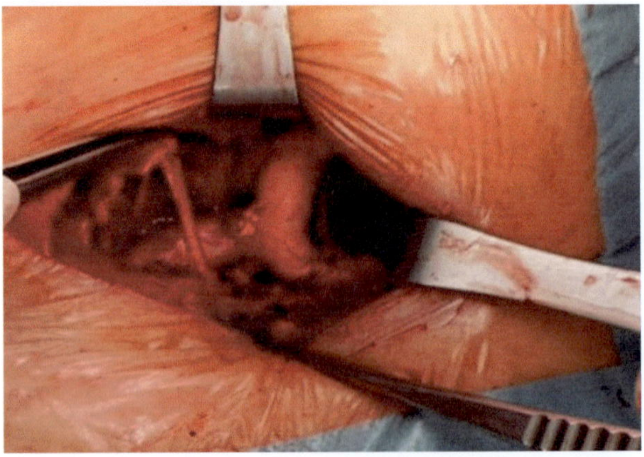

Fig. 11.9 The vertebral artery transposition surgery. V1 segment of the vertebral artery is anastomosed to the common carotid artery

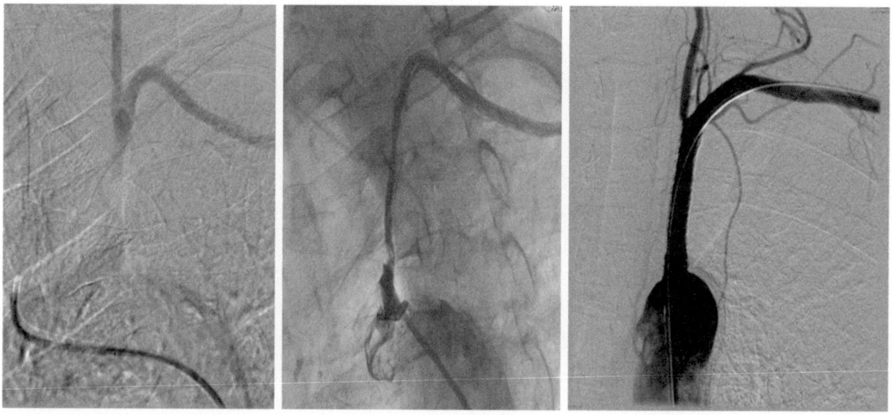

Fig. 11.10 Subclavian steal syndrome. The angiographic catheter was advanced into the brachiocephalic trunk. Retrograde flow was observed through the left vertebral artery, extending into the left arm, indicating occlusion of the left subclavian artery. Using transfemoral access, the occluded left subclavian artery was recanalized with stent deployment, resulting in a successful outcome. After stent placement, the left vertebral artery demonstrated normal anterograde flow

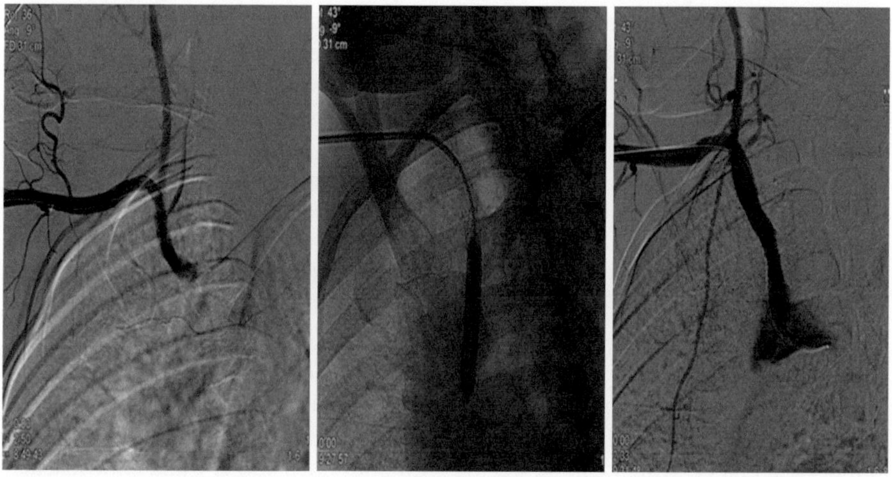

Fig. 11.11 Transradial access. Severe stenosis of the subclavian artery. Predilatation and stent deployment with a satisfactory result

cerebral complications occur in 1–3% of patients treated endovascularly. Additionally, stent fracture, restenosis, and local complications can be observed in approximately 5–7% of cases [6]. Dual antiplatelet therapy is indicated for at least 1–3 months following angioplasty, after which long-term single antiplatelet therapy is recommended. The technical success rate is high, with reported rates of 94% for stenosis and 83% for occlusions. Long-term patency rates are satisfactory, exceeding 70% [7].

11.3.1 Thoracic Outlet Syndrome (TOS)

The subclavian artery, subclavian vein, and the brachial plexus (a large nerve network for the arm) pass through the narrow space at the upper thoracic outlet. Compression of these neurovascular structures can occur due to a hypertrophic cervical rib, an aberrant first rib, tight costoclavicular space, or scalenus muscles. The most common form of TOS is neurogenic TOS, accounting for over 90% of cases [8, 9].

Symptoms of neurogenic TOS include tingling and impaired sensation in the hand, especially when the hand is held in an unfavorable position for extended periods (such as during sleep or while working). Compression of the artery can lead to arm ischemia, particularly when the arm is elevated (as in typists, accordionists, or workers with raised arms). Compression of the subclavian vein and adjacent lymphatic vessels impedes venous and lymphatic return to the heart, potentially causing swelling of the entire arm. Symptoms often worsen with arm elevation (hyperabduction) and deep breathing (inspiration) [8, 9].

Diagnostic tests for TOS may include the Adson, hyperabduction, Roos, and Elvey tests, as well as assessments for Raynaud's phenomenon (e.g., cold water exposure) and, occasionally, electromyography of the upper extremities. Further imaging with Doppler ultrasound, chest X-ray, or computed tomography may be required to identify the presence of a cervical rib or other structural abnormalities.

Neurogenic TOS is typically managed conservatively with physical therapy and medications. Arterial TOS may require surgical intervention, often through supraclavicular or transaxillary approaches, with decompression surgeries tailored to the underlying cause.

Venous TOS is usually treated with anticoagulant medications. There is no strong evidence supporting the use of thrombolysis for thoracic outlet syndrome (TOS). Surgical decompression is rarely indicated for venous TOS [10].

Ischemic stroke in a patient with vertebral artery atherosclerotic stenosis is often more severe and has a higher mortality rate compared to stroke in the carotid circulation. Other less common causes of posterior ischemic symptoms include vasculitis, dissection, trauma, and degenerative osteophyte formation. The estimated prevalence of posterior ischemic stroke is approximately 20–30% [11]. The vertebral artery is divided into four segments (V1–V4). Stenosis most commonly occurs in the V1 segment, which can be treated with both open surgery and endovascular techniques. The other segments of the vertebral artery are more challenging to treat. Surgical reconstruction of the vertebral artery is considered only if medical therapy fails and in patients with severe symptoms such as dizziness, fainting, drop attacks, transient ischemic attacks (TIAs), or stroke.

To plan treatment, imaging studies such as computed tomography (CT) or magnetic resonance angiography (MRA) are essential for diagnosing and evaluating the complete vascular status and vertebral artery dominance. Invasive angiography is used for both diagnosis and as part of endovascular treatment.

Surgical reconstruction of the vertebral artery is indicated in symptomatic cases with >50–60% stenosis when conservative treatment is insufficient. Reconstructive interventions can include:

- **Transposition:** An anastomosis with an adjacent artery, usually the common carotid artery.
- **Bypass Operations:** Using an autogenous graft when transposition is not possible, typically for stenosis in the V3 segment.
- **Decompressive Surgery:** Removal of osteophytes and other abnormal bone-muscular structures, usually in the segment passing through the transverse processes of the spinal vertebrae.

Exposing the vertebral artery is technically demanding due to its deep location, primarily within the intertransverse bone canal. The close proximity to surrounding nerve, venous, arterial, and lymphatic structures further complicates the procedure. Endarterectomy is generally not effective for the vertebral artery; it is used only for the initial part of the vertebral artery in cases such as subclavian steal syndrome. Vertebral artery transposition is considered the most elegant minimally invasive surgical solution, as it is easier, faster, and more reliable compared to autogenous bypass.

Endovascular treatment is a viable option; however, as of now, there is no strong evidence supporting its superiority over conservative management. The decision to pursue endovascular treatment is highly individualized and tailored to each patient's specific needs. Potential complications associated with endovascular treatment include distal embolic events, dissection, stent fracture, restenosis, and local access issues (Figs. 11.12 and 11.13).

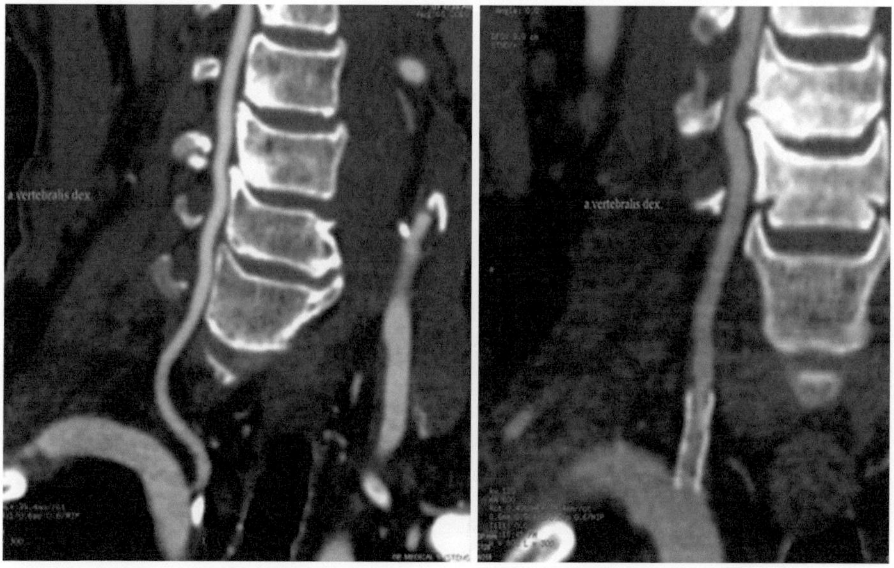

Fig. 11.12 The initial computed tomography scan revealed right subclavian stenosis in a symptomatic patient. Follow-up imaging showed neointimal hyperplasia and restenosis within the stent

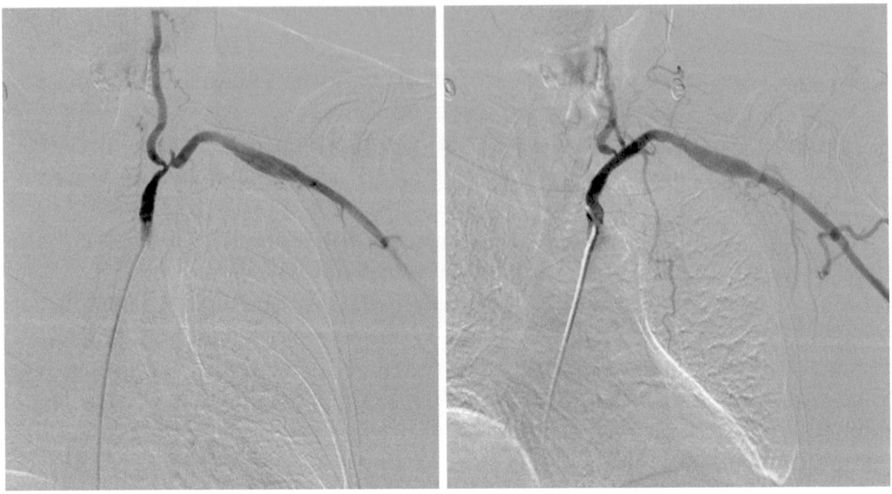

Fig. 11.13 Angiography as part of treatment: In cases of stenosis in the left subclavian artery, which may lead to distal embolic complications affecting the arm and near the origin of the left vertebral artery, stent deployment can potentially impact the flow in the vertebral artery. Therefore, it is crucial to evaluate the entire circle of Willis and the dominance of the vertebral arteries before placing a stent that covers the vertebral artery

References

1. Layton KF, Kallmes DF, Cloft HJ, Lindell EP, Cox VS. Bovine aortic arch variant in humans: clarification of a common misnomer. AJNR Am J Neuroradiol. 2006;27:1541–2.
2. Goray VB, Joshi AR, Garg A, Merchant S, Yadav B, Maheshwari P. Aortic arch variation: a unique case with anomalous origin of both vertebral arteries as additional branches of the aortic arch distal to left subclavian artery. AJNR Am J Neuroradiol. 2005;26:93–5.
3. Takach TJ, Reul GJ, Cooley DA, Duncan JM, Livesay JJ, Gregoric ID, et al. Brachiocephalic reconstruction I: operative and long-term results for complex disease. J Vasc Surg. 2005;42:47–54.
4. Kuhn JE, Lebus VGF, Bible JE. Thoracic outlet syndrome. J Am Acad Orthop Surg. 2015;23:222–32.
5. Ustun C. NEUROwords Dr. Thomas Willis' famous eponym: the circle of Willis. J Hist Neurosci. 2005;14:16–21.
6. Ederle J, Bonati LH, Dobson J, Featherstone RL, Gaines PA, Beard JD, CAVATAS Investigators, et al. Endovascular treatment with angioplasty or stenting versus endarterectomy in patients with carotid artery stenosis in the Carotid and Vertebral Artery Transluminal Angioplasty Study (CAVATAS): long-term follow-up of a randomised trial. Lancet Neurol. 2009;8:898–907.
7. Radak D, Babic S, Sagic D, Tanaskovic S, Kovacevic V, Otasevic P, Rancic Z. Endovascular treatment of symptomatic high-grade vertebral artery stenosis. J Vasc Surg. 2014;60:92–7.
8. Rinehardt EK, Scarborough JE, Bennett KM. Current practice of thoracic outlet decompression surgery in the United States. J Vasc Surg. 2017;66:858–65.
9. Doneddu PE, Coraci D, De Franco P, Paolasso I, Caliandro P, Padua L. Thoracic outlet syndrome: wide literature for few cases. Status of the art. Neurol Sci. 2017;38:383–8.
10. Kearon C, Akl EA, Ornelas J, Blaivas A, Jimenez D, Bounameaux H, Huisman M, et al. Antithrombotic therapy for VTE disease. Chest. 2016;149:315–52.
11. Flossmann E, Rothwell PM. Prognosis of vertebrobasilar transient ischaemic attack and minor stroke. Brain. 2003;126:1940–54.

MIX
Papier aus verantwortungsvollen Quellen
Paper from responsible sources
FSC® C105338

If you have any concerns about our products,
you can contact us on
ProductSafety@springernature.com

In case Publisher is established outside the EU,
the EU authorized representative is:
Springer Nature Customer Service Center GmbH
Europaplatz 3, 69115 Heidelberg, Germany

Printed by Libri Plureos GmbH
in Hamburg, Germany